THE MASSEY LECTURES SERIES

The Massey Lectures are co-sponsored by CBC Radio, House of Anansi Press, and Massey College in the University of Toronto. The series was created in honour of the Right Honourable Vincent Massey, former Governor General of Canada, and was inaugurated in 1961 to provide a forum on radio where major contemporary thinkers could address important issues of our time.

This book comprises the 2018 Massey Lectures, "All Our Relations: Finding the Path Forward," broadcast in November 2018 as part of CBC Radio's *Ideas* series. The producer of the series was Philip Coulter; the executive producer was Greg Kelly.

THE ATKINSON FELLOWSHIP IN PUBLIC POLICY

The Atkinson Fellowship in Public Policy provides a seasoned Canadian journalist with the financial means to pursue a year-long investigation into a critical public policy issue. This award was established by the Atkinson Foundation, the Honderich Family, and the *Toronto Star* in 1988. As a public policy advocate, grant-maker, and investor, Atkinson has promoted social and economic justice in Ontario since 1942.

TANYA TALAGA

Tanya Talaga is the acclaimed author of *Seven Fallen Feathers*, which was the winner of the RBC Taylor Prize, the Shaughnessy Cohen Prize for Political Writing, and the First Nation Communities Read: Young Adult/Adult Award; a finalist for the Hilary Weston Writers' Trust Nonfiction Prize and the BC National Award for Nonfiction; CBC's Nonfiction Book of the Year, a *Globe and Mail* Top 100 Book, and a national bestseller. For more than twenty years, Talaga was a journalist at the *Toronto Star* and is now a columnist at the *Globe and Mail*. She has been nominated five times for the Michener Award in public service journalism, and she was the 2017–18 Atkinson Fellow in Public Policy. Talaga is of Polish and Indigenous descent. Her great-grandmother Liz Gauthier was a residential school survivor. Her great-grandfather Russell Bowen was an Ojibwe trapper and labourer. Her grandmother is a member of Fort William First Nation. Her mother was raised in Raith and Graham, Ontario. Talaga lives in Toronto with her two teenage children.

Also by the Author

Seven Fallen Feathers

ALL OUR RELATIONS

Finding the Path Forward

TANYA TALAGA

ANANSI

Published in Canada and the USA in 2018 by House of Anansi Press Inc.
www.houseofanansi.com

House of Anansi Press is committed to protecting our natural environment.
This book is made of material from well-managed FSC®-certified forests,
recycled materials, and other controlled sources.

House of Anansi Press is a Global Certified Accessible™ (GCA by Benetech)
publisher. The ebook version of this book meets stringent accessibility
standards and is available to students and readers with print disabilities.

25 24 23 22 21   5 6 7 8 9

Library and Archives Canada Cataloguing in Publication

Talaga, Tanya, author
All our relations : finding the path forward / Tanya Talaga.

(CBC Massey lectures)
Includes bibliographical references and index.
Issued in print and electronic formats.
ISBN 978-1-4870-0573-3 (softcover).—ISBN 978-1-4870-0575-7 (EPUB).—
ISBN 978-1-4870-0576-4 (Kindle)

1. Native youth—Suicidal behavior—Canada. 2. Native peoples—Suicidal
behavior—Canada. 3. Native youth—Suicidal behavior—Canada—Prevention.
4. Native peoples—Suicidal behavior—Canada—Prevention. 5. Native youth—
Mental health—Canada. 6. Native peoples—Mental health—Canada. 7. Native
youth—Mental health services—Canada. 8. Native peoples—Mental health
services—Canada. I. Title. II. Series: CBC Massey lectures series

E98.S9T35 2018   362.2808350971   C2018-901983-2
                      C2018-901984-0

Library of Congress Control Number: 2018940369
U.S. ISBN: 978-1-4870-0574-0

Cover design: Alysia Shewchuk
Text design: Ingrid Paulson

*House of Anansi Press respectfully acknowledges that the land on which we
operate is the Traditional Territory of many Nations, including the Anishinabeg,
the Wendat, and the Haudenosaunee. It is also the Treaty Lands of the
Mississaugas of the Credit.*

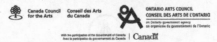

*We acknowledge for their financial support of our publishing program the Canada
Council for the Arts, the Ontario Arts Council, and the Government of Canada.*

Printed and bound in Canada

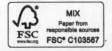

For my sister, nimisenh,
Donna Warren
(1960–2015)

CONTENTS

To the person who is struggling at this moment:

We can choose to continue to think of ourselves as victims and always look to justify our own fears and inadequacies and our own failings by blaming colonialism, or residential schools, or government paternalism, or other realities of our past.

We can also decide, if we choose to do so, that this is a way of thinking that is no longer useful for us as we look to the future.

These factors were certainly part of our past, but it is a past which we have struggled to overcome, and the reality is that we have overcome them.

It is no longer useful for us as individuals, as communities, and ultimately as a Nation to remain stuck in a way of thinking which does not reflect the possibilities for the future.

Matthew Coon Come
Grand Chief, Grand Council of the Crees
(1987–1999, 2009–2017)
The People's Inquiry, Mushkegowuk Council, 2016

....

But don't say in the years to come that you would have lived your life differently if only you had heard this story.

You've heard it now.

Thomas King
The Truth About Stories: A Native Narrative
CBC Massey Lectures, 2003

ONE

WE WERE ALWAYS HERE

IN THE SPRING OF 2017, I was driving down May Street in Thunder Bay, Ontario, with Ricki Strang. We had just gone on an emotional walk along the McIntyre River, which weaves around a strip mall, past a parking lot, and underneath an overpass. We were remembering his younger brother Reggie, whose body was found in the water there on November 1, 2007. Reggie was one of seven First Nations students who died while attending high school in Thunder Bay between 2000 and 2011. Ricki was only sixteen when he woke up in the river on October 26, 2007, the last night he saw his fifteen-year-old brother alive. Ricki mentioned that he had to leave the next day so he could attend a memorial service for Amy Owen, a girl back home in Poplar Hill First Nation, a remote fly-in reserve more than six hundred kilometres northwest of Thunder Bay. He quietly told me that she was really young and that she had died by suicide.

On the evening of January 8, 2017, Amy Owen ran out of her Ottawa-area group home and headed straight for the train tracks across the street. This was where the thirteen-year-old planned to die. The head of the Beacon Home remembers that in the evenings, Amy would talk about how she needed to do it. She wrote it on the walls, on pieces of paper. "I need out of here" was one message. "I want to die" was another.[1] The night that Amy ran, staff at the seven-bed facility for teenage girls were ready and right behind her. Amy would not be successful that day.

One of Amy's closest friends would be: that same night, more than one thousand kilometres away, in the remote Northern Ontario fly-in First Nations community of Wapekeka, twelve-year-old Jolynn Winter took her own life.

Two days later, on January 10, also in Wapekeka, Sandra Fox stepped out briefly to get pain relievers for the persistent discomfort in her leg. When she came home, she found that her daughter, Chantell

Fox, also twelve years old and Jolynn's best friend, had hanged herself.

Amy would follow suit, but not for another three months.

Seven girls in all, whose lives had intersected back home or in group homes or care facilities far away from their First Nations communities, took their lives within a year of one another.

Alayna Moose, twelve. Kanina Sue Turtle, fifteen. Jolynn Winter, twelve. Chantell Fox, twelve. Amy Owen, thirteen. Jenera Roundsky, twelve. Jeannie Grace Brown, thirteen.

Far beyond the dense, brightly lit skyscrapers and condominiums in the cities that ring the Great Lakes of southern Ontario, the people of Nishnawbe Aski Nation (NAN), a political organization comprising forty-nine First Nations spread out over the northern two-thirds of the province, have been trying to stop their children from dying.[2]

The seven girls were from Poplar Hill First Nation and Wapekeka First Nation, both communities with populations of less than five hundred people. The anguish over the loss of the girls blankets NAN territory, covering the land east from the Manitoba border to James Bay, and then north to the shallow shores of Hudson Bay. The deaths of Jolynn and Chantell — granddaughter of Wapekeka's chief, Brennan Sainnawap — hit the community so hard that nearly all the teenagers living there were put on suicide watch. Counsellors and mental health experts from the cities were flown in, and distraught children were sent on medical flights to be assessed by psychiatrists and doctors in southern hospitals, far away from home. The sadness overwhelmed the tiny, tight-knit community.[3]

Some people have called the deaths of the seven girls a "suicide pact," implying that the action was designed and formulated as a grand plan. Anna Betty Achneepineskum, former deputy grand chief of NAN, bristles at that term. She sees things differently. It was not a pact; that word covers up the root of the problem — what the girls were experiencing was tremendous grief, and as a result they were struggling to cope.

"Kids don't talk about suicide or talk about a pact for no reason," says Anna Betty. "They are talking to each other about their trauma. And in a small community, you just can't isolate yourself from trauma."[4]

It did not have to be this way. In the early summer of 2017, six months before his granddaughter's death, Chief Sainnawap sent a note to Health

Canada, the federal bureaucracy in charge of health funding for all the Indigenous people in the country, begging for assistance. The community leaders had discovered that some of their youth had made a suicide pact. The leaders were seeking $376,706 to immediately hire a mental health team of four workers who could deliver prevention and intervention programs and help create a healthy community environment.[5] The request was denied. When the girls' deaths made national and international news, the community later heard through the Canadian Broadcasting Corporation that Wapekeka's request had come at an "awkward time" during the budgetary cycle — there simply wasn't any funding available.[6]

This was not the first time that a cry for help from the community was ignored. In 2015, after twenty-two years, Ottawa abruptly cut the funding for the annual Survivors of Suicide Conference in Wapekeka, where there had been sixteen deaths by suicide from 1982 to 1999.[7] Wapekeka and the surrounding First Nations had grown to rely on the annual meeting as a time to come together in an Indigenous space, honour those they had lost, and together seek a new path forward. The conference meant much to the people who had lived the experience of loss and who couldn't afford a charter plane to a big-city, Western-focused medical conference on the issue.

On January 18, 2017, days after NAN Grand Chief Alvin Fiddler had flown to Wapekeka to attend the funerals of Chantell and Jolynn, he got on another plane in Thunder Bay, Ontario, and flew to the nation's capital. There he held a news conference at the National Press Gallery with Joshua Frogg, Wapekeka's band manager and Chantell's uncle; Sioux Lookout's Dr. Michael Kirlew; National Chief of the Assembly of First Nations Perry Bellegarde; Charlie Angus, a New Democratic Party member of Parliament; and Jonathan Solomon, the grand chief of the Mushkegowuk Council of Cree Nations along the western side of James Bay. The council's eight communities had suffered unbearably high numbers of youth suicides and attempts — six hundred attempts alone since 2009, so many that it prompted them to hold their own two-year-long "People's Inquiry into Our Suicide Pandemic." Nearly three hundred people from the community had participated, seventy-seven personal stories were recorded, and recommendations were made in a report released in January 2016.[8] By the time of the news conference, exactly one year later, the council still had not received a response from the federal government.

In February 2016, a few weeks after the release of the Mushkegowuk report, Fiddler and NAN had declared a "state of emergency" — NAN territory was experiencing a health and suicide crisis. Children were dying from preventable illnesses and by their own hands because of a lack of access to proper nursing and medical care. In May 2014, five-year-old Brody Meekis, from Sandy Lake First Nation, died of strep throat — an illness that can be cured with antibiotics if properly diagnosed.[9] Brody had been at the Sandy Lake nursing station with his two brothers; all were feeling unwell, but the boys were sent home without having had throat swab tests. Instead, they were told to use Vicks VapoRub and come back if the symptoms persisted. Because they didn't have a car and couldn't access the sole medical transport van at Sandy Lake, they were unable to return to the nursing station for further treatment. When Brody's father tried to get another appointment, he was told a time wasn't available for at least a week. Brody continued to get worse. Days later, his mother took him back to the nursing station, but it was too late. He passed away.[10] Brody was the second child in NAN territory to die of strep throat, a common, treatable infection.[11] For NAN, Brody's death highlighted a host of issues with the poorly supported health clinics on reserves: a lack of doctors and adequate staffing, issues with nurses' qualifications, a shortage of supplies, and the infrastructure of the clinics themselves being below standards.

NAN had outlined a series of directives that had to be executed within ninety days in order to manage the state of emergency. At the time, these were ignored.

So, too, were the mental health recommendations drawn from the inquest following the deaths of the Seven Fallen Feathers: NAN high school students Jethro Anderson, Curran Strang, Paul Panacheese, Robyn Harper, Reggie Bushie, Kyle Morrisseau, and Jordan Wabasse. Between 2000 and 2011, all seven lost their lives while attending high school in Thunder Bay. Because their communities did not have basic functioning high schools, the children had to move six hundred kilometres away from their mothers and fathers, their sisters and brothers, their homes and their communities, in order to pursue their education. Made on June 28, 2016, the inquest's recommendations — specifically numbers thirty-seven and thirty-eight — addressed the suicide crisis. Recommendation number thirty-seven called on the federal and provincial governments to work with NAN to devise a mental health plan for youth, and recommendation number thirty-eight called for the Province of Ontario to "improve consistency and enhance co-ordination" of on-reserve mental health services. At the time, those two recommendations were also ignored.[12]

Alvin Fiddler had had enough. The father of two teenage girls and the son of Moses Fiddler — a witness to the signing of the 1929 adhesion to Treaty No. 9, which saw much of what is now Northwestern Ontario swallowed by the Crown — Alvin was frustrated and tired of working within the government's parameters and antiquated legislation. For years he had been playing by the government's rules, following the proper protocol channels. NAN was constantly financing studies, writing reports, and applying for funding to the federal government so that its communities could receive basic services such as clean, drinkable water, proper sewage treatment, working fire trucks, and police services. Progress was always woefully slow, if any was made at all. Too often, it was only when First Nations deaths were reported in the news that the government took action.

The day before Fiddler started the press conference on January 19, 2017, NAN released a searing letter he had written to Prime Minister Justin Trudeau, who had promised in December 2015 to "reset" Canada's relationship with Indigenous people, establishing a "renewed, nation-to-nation relationship with First Nations peoples, one that understands that the constitutionally guaranteed rights of First Nations in Canada are not an inconvenience but rather a sacred obligation."[13]

Fiddler's letter described how fundamentally broken the relationship was between NAN communities and the Government of Canada. It outlined a devastating list of all the unacted-upon court orders, the ignored inquest findings, and Indigenous and Northern Affairs Canada's consistent failure to respond in times of crisis — all during Trudeau's brief tenure in office.

"As you have acknowledged in the House of Commons," Fiddler wrote, "these tragedies are a result of our colonial history, and we need to fix a relationship that has broken over the past decade, and indeed over centuries between Canada and Indigenous peoples. We are Treaty partners. But, this partnership changed over time, increasingly defined by choice on one side, and legislative constraints on the other.

"First Nations are not sitting on their hands and expecting the federal government to solve the tragedies of their communities. But, we have been legislated into a position where our power is to make proposals and seek program dollars from your bureaucracy. When we are then ignored, our hands are tied and our children continue to needlessly die."[14]

THE TRAGEDY OF SUICIDE is that it is preventable. Each life gone is a lost opportunity for someone to have received help. The scope of the suicide problem is immense. From 1986 through December 2017, there were more than 558 suicides across NAN territory, a community comprising only forty-nine thousand people. Last year, 2017, was the worst in recent memory, with thirty-seven suicides. Most of the suicides are by hanging, and the majority are by young men. The number of attempts — those who try to take their lives but fail — is even greater. Since 1986, an almost incomprehensible eighty-eight children between the ages of ten and fourteen have killed themselves.[15]

The high youth-suicide numbers are not just

found in NAN territory. According to the Centre for Suicide Prevention, in Canada suicide and self-inflicted injuries are the leading causes of death for First Nations youth and adults up to the age of forty-four. The centre also reports that the suicide rate for young First Nations men between the ages of fifteen and twenty-four is 126 per 100,000, compared to 24 per 100,000 for non-Indigenous young men. First Nations women have a suicide rate of 35 per 100,000, compared to 5 per 100,000 for non-Indigenous women.[16]

Suicide among Inuit is even more pronounced. Jack Hicks is an adjunct professor at the University of Saskatchewan in community health and epidemiology and a former suicide prevention advisor for the Government of Nunavut and Inuit Tapiriit Kanatami, a national organization protecting and advancing the rights of Inuit in Canada. He says that for the past fifteen years, the Inuit suicide rate has been ten times the national average.[17]

Indigenous youth suicide is not just a Canadian problem. Across the globe, Indigenous people living in colonized countries share a crushing commonality: their children are dying by their own hands. While there is no global data on how many Indigenous children and youth are taking their own lives, the statistics gathered from colonized nations point to similarities. The first is that suicide is a modern phenomenon within Indigenous Nations. In Canada, before the forced resettlement of Inuit people off the land and into towns, and before the Indian Residential Schools, suicide was uncommon. This also holds true for the Sami population in Scandinavia and the Indigenous people in Brazil and in Australia. And in each of these colonized countries, Indigenous young men have among the highest suicide rates globally.

Nearly one in three Sami have thought about or attempted suicide, says Jon Petter Stoor, a Sami psychologist and project manager of the Sami Norwegian National Advisory Board on Mental Health and Substance Abuse (SANKS).[18] In the United States, Native Americans take their lives anywhere from three to ten times the national average. In 2015, the Oglala Sioux Pine Ridge Reservation in South Dakota declared a state of emergency when fourteen youths took their own lives within a seven-month period between August 2014 and April 2015.[19] The state of Amazonas in Brazil comprises 30 percent of Brazil's Indigenous lands, and Indigenous people make up 4.8 percent of the state's population of 3.5 million, but they account for 19 percent of all suicides.[20] In Guarani-Kaiowá, a community of thirty-one thousand in southwestern Brazil, the suicide rate is thirty-four times higher within the Indigenous population than among the non-Indigenous population. Most die by hanging, and most are young.[21]

Australia continues to struggle with suicide among the Aboriginal people and the Indigenous people of the Torres Strait Islands. Aboriginals are the original inhabitants of the mainland and the island of Tasmania. Torres Strait Islanders are the First Peoples of the Torres Strait Islands, located between Papua New Guinea and Cape York Peninsula in the state of Queensland. In 2016, 162 Indigenous people in Australia took their own lives. Suicides account for 5.5 percent of all Aboriginal deaths, compared to 1.7 percent in the non-Indigenous population. From 2012 to 2016, intentional self-harm was the leading cause of death for all Aboriginal people between the ages of fifteen and thirty-four, and it was the second leading cause of death for those between the ages of thirty-five and forty-four.[22]

In a groundbreaking 2006 study titled "Aboriginal and Torres Strait Islander Suicide in Context," Dr. Ernest Hunter and Dr. Helen Milroy, the first Aboriginal psychiatrist in Australia, point out that self-harm was once uncommon within Indigenous communities in Australia; now it is the norm. Many children are exposed to suicide or suicidal behaviour. They are part of the first generation of children whose early development is regularly exposed to the "threat or act of self-annihilation."[23]

There is a narrative, a shared history of all colonized people: trauma, exposure to suicidal tendencies when young, a history of discriminatory legislation and policies, and a lack of psycho-cultural identity. Milroy says the complex interplay of all these factors and so many more is unique to each lived experience. For Indigenous peoples, underlying that life experience is the reality of genocide: "We have come from a history of genocide, and genocide is about the deliberate annihilation of a race; it is about wanting to remove us from the Earth permanently, which is very different as a concept from transgenerational trauma. It is trauma on a more massive scale — psychologically, physically, spiritually, culturally. It is another level of trauma again."

Indigenous children and youth are born under the staggering weight of history: the historical injustices of colonization; the forced removal off the land by extermination or segregation; the cultural genocide effected by government policy and religious indoctrination; the intergenerational trauma stemming from years of poverty, abuse, and identity oppression. They are more often than not displaced, suffering from economic, social, and cultural marginalization that can trigger substance abuse and violence. They are caught between historical and what the United Nations calls "present-day dynamics."[24]

Generations of Indigenous children have grown up largely in communities without access to the basic determinants of health — income and social status, access to clean water and air, safe houses and communities, supportive families and a connection to their traditions, and access to a basic education and health care services — even in a country like Canada, revered around the world for its fresh water, high living standards, education system, and public health care. According to the World Health Organization, a people's health is the direct result of its social, political, and environmental circumstances. Children are not in control of their determinants of health. They are born into them.[25]

In Indigenous communities, the lasting impact of colonial history has resulted in the near absence of these determinants of health. It has also directly resulted in a severing of the crucial spiritual, emotional, and physical tethers to the past. The historical separation of Indigenous people from their land, the separation of children from their parents, the separation from their traditional culture and ways of living — all of these things have contributed to a spiritual emptiness that has resulted in generations of children's deaths. This book is about righting past wrongs; it is about collectively upholding and adhering to the rights of Indigenous children — the right to proper health care, an equitable education, clean drinking water, a secure community, and a warm, safe home to sleep in at night, tucked in by parents who tell them that they love them. It is about restoring their pride in who they are and where they come from.

THERE ARE FOUR QUESTIONS every Indigenous person must answer in order to understand who they are. According to Senator Murray Sinclair, the first First Nations justice in the province of Manitoba and chairman of the Indian Residential Schools Truth and Reconciliation Commission in Canada from 2009 to 2015, those questions are: Where do

I come from? Where am I going? What is my purpose? Who am I?[26]

Traditionally, all Indigenous Nations have a deep connection to the land. They believe human beings are part of a greater life story, part of a continuum of all life on Earth, and that each individual being plays their own role as a custodian, safeguarding the land for the next generation. Every person born has a purpose, every person belongs.

In his landmark 2003 Massey Lectures titled *The Truth About Stories*, the award-winning author and scholar Thomas King deconstructs the colonial and post-colonial narrative imposed upon Indigenous people by settlers in North America. Before the arrival of Christopher Columbus in 1492, the Indigenous people of Turtle Island, or North America, were often cast as "Noble Savages," mildly docile creatures of nature enjoying the "terrestrial paradise" of Mother Earth.[27] Written accounts of early explorers and settlers bolster those sentiments — Indigenous men wore loincloths and painted their faces with strong colours, and everyone lived in large communal families. According to those first observers, the people they encountered were godless pagans, living in the bush, completely uncivilized by the standards of early Western Judeo-Christian society.

This image of "natural man," untouched by civilization, continued to preoccupy European intellectuals during the seventeenth- and eighteenth-century Enlightenment period.[28] In the nineteenth century, the theory of social Darwinism was used to justify hierarchies of class, race, and ethnicity. The Victorian era took those theories and ran with them, adding in a good dose of the importance of Empire.[29] Fast-forward to the twentieth century, and all the misconceptions of the past were cooked up into an image of the stereotypical Indian wearing a headdress and riding around the prairies on horseback. That image was perpetuated by Hollywood and portrayed by non-Indigenous actors on film and TV. Burt Reynolds reportedly wore a wig to play Navajo Joe in the spaghetti western of the same name. In the movie, he hunts down a bank robber and murderer of an entire tribe, killing him with a tomahawk thrown directly into his forehead. Johnny Depp played Tonto, the ever-present Indian sidekick to the white hero in *The Lone Ranger*. And Tom Laughlin wrote and starred in a number of Billy Jack movies, about a half-breed Navajo who is also a Green Beret Vietnam veteran and a martial arts master. No Indigenous person saw themselves in any of those characters. They weren't real. And yet they became a part of every Indigenous person's reality.

Indigenous people have been trapped in these identity constructs in part because of their near-complete absence from the written narratives of the colonist nations. In Canada, for example, the history of the Indian Residential School system was excluded from school curricula for generations, leaving the majority of the population unaware of Indigenous experiences of parent–child separation and forced assimilation. People often tell me that they wish they had known what was happening inside the walls of those 139 Indian Residential Schools, where an estimated six thousand Indigenous children died because they were being mistreated, abused, neglected, or starved; that they didn't really understand the effects of the trauma endured by the students when they left school, and the subsequent trauma then passed on to the students' family members and children.

In Thomas King's analysis of the advent of contemporary Indigenous writers, such as Haisla author Eden Robinson, Kiowa author N. Scott Momaday, and Ojibwe writer and painter Ruby

Slipperjack, he notes that, with few exceptions, "Contemporary Native writers have shown little interest in using the past as a setting, preferring instead to place their fictions in the present."

> What Native writers discovered, I believe, was that the North American past, the one that had been created in novels and histories, the one that had been heard on radio and seen on theatre screens and on television, the one that had been part of every school curriculum for the last two hundred years, that past was unusable, for it had not only trapped Native people in a time warp, it also insisted that our past was all we had.
> No present.
> No future.
> And to believe in such a past is to be dead.[30]

Where do we come from?
There is a rich history, one that is not often widely published or discussed in mainstream education and discourse, but it has always been there. And these stories are passed down by Elders to subsequent generations. Elders are the knowledge keepers of ceremonies, rites, and laws — traditions that form the core of a society's culture, history, and

identity. Elders remind us who we are and where we need to go.[31]

In 2006, Dr. Jim Dumont gave the inaugural Newbery Lecture at the University of Sudbury. Dumont is the chief of the Eastern Doorway of the Three Fires Midewiwin Lodge. The Midewiwin is the Grand Medicine Society of the Anishinabeg people. While this explanation does not do them complete justice, its members can be compared to a grand council of Elders who are in charge of safe-keeping and teaching the most sacred stories — the stories of how life came to be, and how one should conduct and live one's life.

"My real name, my spirit name, is Onaubinisay," Dumont begins. He tells the audience that he is originally from a place called Shawanaga First Nation, which is around the central Georgian Bay–Parry Sound area, and that he is of the Waubizhayshee Ododaim (Marten clan). This is his identity — this is who he is.[32]

He continues to tell the story of his life as a scholar and a teacher. In 1967, Dumont became one of the first graduates of the University of Sudbury, and in 1970 he completed his master's degree at the University of Toronto. Instead of pursuing a career in academia, he instead chose to move back to Manitoulin Island, where he could focus his studies on his own culture's history and traditions. It was during this time that he was approached by Dr. J. W. Edward Newbery, after whom the lecture is named.[33] Newbery was a minister of the United Church of Canada, and from 1960 to 1967 he was the president and principal of Huntington College. In 1970, he founded the Institute of Indian Studies at the University of Sudbury.[34]

Dumont recounts that Dr. Newbery asked him to teach in the department. Dumont resisted — he didn't feel he had a strong enough grasp of Indigenous knowledge. Dr. Newbery continued to pursue him. Four years later, Dumont finally felt capable enough in his understanding of Indigenous culture and traditions to pass the knowledge on to others. What resulted was a department of Indigenous Studies that was completely unique in the country at the time, perhaps even in the world.

"It's the only program that puts tradition, culture, our own ways, our own history, our own teachings, our own knowledge, our own spirituality and our own language at the very core of everything that we do," Dumont says. But he also acknowledges that the program had limitations, as it remained "within the boundaries of the western educational institution."[35]

The lecture, titled "Indigenous Intelligence," centres around a very important question: "Are we really speaking from our own Indigenous knowledge or have we become anthropologists and ethnologists of our own traditions, our own cultures?" It is to this paradigm that Dumont has dedicated his life's work: defining, building, and exercising Indigenous Intelligence, unhindered by the Western worldview.

"The very first concept at the centre of everything is the spirit," he says. "I am a spirit who is walking through this world. That is who Anishinabe is."

From there, he tells the story of his people, of the Ojibwe, my mother and grandmother's people. The Ojibwe are part of the greater Anishinabeg people — the Odawa, the Potawatomi, the Oji-Cree, and the Algonquin — who historically have lived along Gichigami, or Lake Superior, and the surrounding Great Lakes area.

Dumont describes how "In the beginning, there was only darkness — darkness because there was yet not light; silence because there was nothing to make a sound... It was a time, not of nothingness, but a time when there was nothing yet that had come into being." He explains how the Spirit, or Creator, came into being from this nothingness and "the unconscious becomes conscious." The Spirit wanted to know his own thought and see it reflected back, so the Spirit sent a "seed thought" out into the darkness, where it left a bright imprint in the sky, and that was a star. The starry night was created and formed by the Creator's thoughts. So, too, was the Earth, and from the Earth the Creator made human beings.

Thereafter, the Spirit created the universe by forming a circle from heart and mind. The circle is a fundamental concept of Indigenous Intelligence, underscoring how everything is interrelated and life operates in a circular pattern. Central to life in the Indigenous worldview is relationship. Being of the Earth, we are connected to the Earth. Being of the Spirit, we are connected to the Spirit — and to each other.

This is in contrast to the Western worldview. Judeo-Christianity puts human beings at the top of the hierarchy of the creation story. This view is reinforced by evolutionary theory, which sees humans as the ultimate evolutionary achievement. Western thinking also tends to be linear, not cyclical, and it is often filtered through the lens of psychology and science, the rational over the spiritual. As a consequence, Indigenous people have been forced to measure up to a definition of intelligence that undermines and devalues their culture, tradition, history, and knowledge.

It is this exact issue, this tension between Indigenous Knowledge and the Western worldview, that inspired Johan Turi, a traditional reindeer herder and wolf hunter, to write *Turi's Book of Lappland*, published in 1910. Turi, who was at the time around fifty years old, was the first Sami author to publish a secular book in the Sami language. The Danish translator Emilie Demant Hatt, who first met Turi in 1904 and lived with him in order to help him write the book, observed that Turi blamed lack of knowledge of the Sami way of life as "the root of all evil that has befallen them at the hands of the settlers...He saw that if things continued in this way the end would be death and destruction for the race to which he belonged, and whose life he led."[36]

For thousands of years, the Sami people have lived in the northern regions of Finland, Norway, Sweden, and Russia, an area known in the Western world as "Lapland" but which the original Indigenous people call Sápmi. They are united by their linguistic heritage (nine languages across the four countries) and by their cultural, social, and economic links, central to which is reindeer herding.[37]

Turi begins by declaring: "I am a Lapp* who, throughout my life, have busied myself with all manner of Lapp work, and I know all about Lapp life. I have heard tell that the Swedish Government will help us all they can, but they don't really understand our life and circumstances, because no Lapp can explain it to them...Now I've thought that it would be a good thing if there was a book which told everything about Lapp life and circumstances so that folk didn't have to keep asking...'What are Lapps' circumstances?'"[38]

He says that in the beginning, the Sami lived a peaceful, idyllic life by the sea. "No one has heard that the Lapps came to this land from any other place. From the very earliest times they have been up here in Lappland."

They lived off fish and wild game, and eventually they came to follow the reindeer, relying on them for most things in their lives, from eating

---

* Until about 1980, almost all non-Sami people referred to the Sami as "Lapp," a term now considered derogatory; its usage was discouraged as far back as the Second World War. Neil Kent, *The Sámi Peoples of the North: A Social and Cultural History* (London: C. Hurst, 2014), 11, 19.

the meat to drinking the milk and blood and making cheese. He describes in beautiful detail the existence of the herder, who is less a "nomad" than an expert in seasonal migration patterns, journeying over high mountain ridges in the winter, calving in the late spring, milking reindeer, and even hunting wolves on skis. And he elucidates with great care the traditional life of the Sami: the family structure, the care and schooling of children, the medicinal remedies and treatment of injury and illness.

Forever, the Sami have been at one with the reindeer, says Turi, pointing out that they migrated together, north and south; both are a little shy, and because of that they have both been driven away from their natural lands.

In his descriptions of the Sami life, Turi circles back again and again to contact with settlers, mostly farmers, who were proliferating with the support of the government in order to establish the agricultural sector. He describes how the Sami were pushed out of their traditional grazing lands, both by means of government policy and by physical confrontation: "When folk increased and multiplied in Norway, then they began to hate the Lapps, in some places so badly that they plundered and beat them, and some Lapps they killed, because the Lapps' herds grazed in those places where they had always been accustomed to graze... Now the laws in Norway against the Lapps are like a veil through which the sharpest eye cannot see. And that veil has already made many conditions unsafe for the Lapps."

He describes how the Sami have been pushed to the farthest reaches, the most uninhabitable environments, "where there are no other folk than Lapps, that is on the naked high fells." As a result, the Sami feel like "an unwanted strange dog." His people are powerless, he says. Settlement has caused their destruction; few know where and how to work without the reindeer, so they don't get married, they don't have children. They can no longer see their future.

"And in this there is great suffering," he says, "when the claims of the body must be suppressed, and the love of the heart destroyed, and everyone who thinks over the matter understands this."

At the time, Turi was mocked by his contemporaries, both Sami and non-Sami, who looked upon writing as a waste of time. But it had long been a dream of his to chronicle their life as it was actually lived, "so that folk shouldn't come to twist everything round till the Lapps are always slandered, and always made out to be in the wrong." He also felt that it would be beneficial to his own people, so that they could reflect upon their lives and circumstances. The book, which was translated into ten languages, does not end with a lament. Instead, it leaves the reader with reproductions of Turi's drawings, which further illustrate the seasonal migration of the reindeer and explicate his vivid, intricate, and nuanced portrait of one of the oldest cultures in the world.

THE ABORIGINES SAY they have always been in Australia, that the continent surrounded by what we now call the Indian and Pacific Oceans has always been their home. As Helen Milroy says, "We were always here."

They lived within their own social order, and they proliferated across the continent, learning from the land how to produce crops over tens of thousands of years of careful grooming and farming. When the British arrived to develop a penal colony on Sydney Cove in 1788, explorers noted there were villages of anywhere from one to five thousand people, with houses large enough to accommodate groups of fifty. Stone houses with thatched roofs were also common.[39]

Some of these villages may have been the oldest in the world. A recent analysis of a midden, or garbage pile, found by the Hopkins River in Western Australia dates back eighty thousand years — ten thousand years before the first humans left the African continent.[40]

In Canada, artifacts that go back five thousand years have been discovered along the scenic shores of Lake Ontario. And while it is a subject of debate among academics, some believe that the combined population of North and South America at that time was ninety million Indigenous souls.[41]

Ninety million Indigenous people living in longhouses, wigwams, tipis, or houses in villages and cities. They had their own customs, laws, systems of governance, and cultures. In northern South America, Indigenous Nations developed astrological charts and used them to construct pyramids that formed the centres of city structures. Complex political systems were at the heart of these cities; there were moral codes, monarchs, chieftainships, and even some evidence of the use of democracy before the concept was even talked about in Europe.[42]

Between the years 800 and 1200, on the eastern

half of Turtle Island, near what is now known as St. Louis, a highly evolved city of nearly twenty thousand people called Cahokia was established by the Mississippi. Centred around the third-largest pyramid on the continent, Cahokia was the largest, most advanced city north of the Rio Grande and at the time rivalled in size the city of London, England.

More than two hundred packed-earth pyramids, or mounds, made up Cahokia and the surrounding area. About half were built within a five-square-mile zone designed around the four sacred directions and the upper and lower worlds. The pyramids were surrounded by open plazas, and beyond were thousands of thatched houses, temples, and public spaces.[43] There were complex rings of irrigation and transportation canals and fields of maize. Located at the merging of the Missouri, Illinois, and Mississippi Rivers, the city was also a busy port, attracting traders from many tribes throughout the continent.[44]

In the country of Brazil, it is believed that between one and five million people lived in the Amazon area. More than two hundred "geoglyphs"—geometric figures or designs formed on the ground—have been found in the state of Acre, some as large as the states of Illinois and Indiana put together, suggesting the presence of a complex Indigenous civilization.[45]

The New World, so to speak, was already an Old World.

This realization often runs through my mind as I drive around my neighbourhood, down a street that connects Eastern Avenue and Queen Street East, just on the outskirts of the Beach neighbourhood, on the traditional territory of the Mississaugas of the New Credit First Nation, whose lands encompassed most of modern-day Toronto. The name Mississaugas derives from the Anishinaabemowin *Missisakis*, or "many river mouths." The French called the Ojibwe the Mississaugas, and the name stuck. The Mississaugas were traditionally allied with the Three Fires Council, which is made up of the Ojibwe, the Odawa, and the Potawatomi Nations. The Three Fires Council is one of the oldest political confederacies on Turtle Island and still exists today.[46]

I have driven this road a million times, as has everyone else who lives in the neighbourhood. It isn't more than half a block long, a shortcut running past the McDonald's restaurant, behind the Alliance Atlantic movie theatres and the Swiss Chalet rotisserie, to the liquor store and pet shop on Queen Street East.

In the spring of 2018, this road was given a name: Kichigo Road, after an Ojibwe family who lived in the Beach neighbourhood by Ashbridge's Bay, now the site of some of the most expensive homes in Canada and of Toronto's giant sewage treatment plant. The Keeshig family were here thousands of years before the British arrived, before Toronto was the City of York, and until spring 2018, any notion, any trace of them had been completely erased. The Ashbridges came from Pennsylvania and settled in the area in 1794. For two centuries they lived on one property, where a particularly well-kept historic brick house off Queen Street East now sits. They were also granted six hundred acres for farming, from the lakefront to Danforth Avenue.[47]

When I think about this, Murray Sinclair's words echo in my ears. I wonder: Where do I come from, what is my purpose, where do I belong?

I am a single mother of two children. My father was a proud Polish Canadian and my mother grew up in the bush, on the traditional lands of Fort William First Nation, where the waters divide on the back of the Turtle's shell. She grew up in a place where there was no plumbing, no bathroom, in a cabin on land her family did not own but had lived near or on for as long as anyone can remember.

My mother was raised by her grandmother, a residential school survivor who would not allow Anishinaabemowin to be spoken in her home, because at residential school she had been taught that everything Indian was dirty. If my mother's grandfather wanted to speak the language, he had to go outside. He was a labourer and a trapper who, according to family lore, had fled residential school. I remember that the floors of the tipi I played in as a child, on the land near the cabin, were lined with soft, black bear fur, and there was always plenty of fresh fish to eat.

My mother's three brothers — Maurice, Bill, and Alvie — were in the child welfare system, gone from us. I did not know my mother had any brothers until I was in my twenties. That was when they found us. That was when my uncle Maurice called my grandmother Margaret and asked if she was his mother. That was when two of them — brave and kind Maurice; and handsome Bill, with his jet-black hair styled just like Elvis's — came home. But we lost Alvie, who died in the United States after living his life as a travelling carnival hand.

My mother gave my sister, Debbie, up for adoption after taking care of her for one year, because she wanted a better life for her daughter, a life she knew she could not provide as a teenage mother. Debbie was raised in Manitoba by a family who changed her name to Donna. I met my sister when I was twenty-four or twenty-five. I had the joy of listening to her laugh and seeing her flash the exact same smile I have seen cross my mother's face thousands of times. But we did not have her for long. We lost her on May 7, 2015, to a sudden heart attack.

I grew up here in the city, in a cookie-cutter subdivision, disconnected from my mother's ancestors, a by-product of the residential school system and the Indian Act, but always aware of trying to reclaim what was lost for the next generation.

Aaniin. Boozhoo.
Tanya Talaga Ndishnikaaz.
Aaniin ezhinikaazoyan?
Aandi wenjibaayan?[48]

Hello, greetings.
My name is Tanya Talaga.
What is your name?
Where are you from?
Where do you belong?

TWO

BIG BROTHER'S HUNGER

LISTEN.

When Edmund Metatawabin gifts you with a story, you had better listen.

Ed is standing on his homemade raft, a sixteen-by-sixty-three-foot colossus slowly making its way down the swollen Albany River, a remote 982-kilometre waterway that begins in Northwestern Ontario and feeds into James Bay. The raft, made by Ed's own hands, is just giant cedar logs lying side by side and tied together with generous loops of rope. On top of the raft, taking up about half of its platform, is a small wooden cabin that resembles a motor home. Inside the cabin you can hear muffled laughter, dishes clanking, and the sweet smell of warm bannock.

I'm standing beside him in my brown rainsuit, covered from head to toe in revolutionary fabric advertised to keep anyone dry in any conditions. But the high-priced suit from the city has become damp under the weight of the water that the clouds are scooping up from the Albany and pelting at us with all their might.

The driving rain is pummelling Ed's brown construction jacket; bits of light from inside the cabin reflect off the orange safety tape on his coat.

Ed turns to me and says, "Big Brother is always hungry."

Big Brother has an insatiable appetite, a relentless hunger that rises up from his grumbling belly and makes him a voracious monster. His massive jaws never stop chomping; his mouth moves like a giant sawmill, devouring anything that comes his way.

Big Brother is so hungry that he has turned his Little Brother into a slave, tasked with heading out into the vast wilderness to find him food. So Little Brother ventures out alone into the northern forests, walking among the scaly-looking red-barked tamarack trees that line the dark waters of the meandering rivers that bleed into the giant bays in the north and to the east. Little Brother walks through the black spruce, which have grown tall and lean back from the cold wind blowing along the river's edge. As he goes, Little Brother chops down everything that he sees. He gathers everything up in large bundles so he can take it all back to Big Brother to feed his hungry belly.

Little Brother does not just gather wood. He also sweeps up all the fish from the black rivers, and he steals the gold and the diamonds from deep, deep inside the Earth's crust.

"Cruel Big Brother. He eats and he eats and he eats," Ed says as water drips off his oilskin fedora.[1]

Ed is a community leader to his people, the Cree of James Bay. He is a survivor and the man in charge of what we lovingly call our "cruise down the Albany."

Ed was one of the 150,000 Indigenous Canadians who were separated from their parents and sent to residential schools. From the mid-1880s to 1996 there were 139 church-run and government-funded residential schools across Canada, 17 in Ontario. The schools' purpose was to convert children to Christianity and isolate them from their homes, families, traditions, and culture, in order to assimilate them to the Canadian way of life.

At the age of seven, Ed was taken from his

family and sent to the notorious St. Anne's Indian Residential School, run by the Oblate Catholic nuns in Fort Albany, on the James Bay coast. There he was physically assaulted regularly and sexually abused by one of the staff members. He and his fellow inmates often went to bed hungry, and they lived in fear of the homemade electric chair used to punish the children. Survivors report students being strapped to the chair and electrocuted until they were semiconscious.[2]

Ed left St. Anne's a broken teenage boy, and when he returned home, he was a stranger to his parents, his siblings, and his Cree culture. He took off, heading out west, where he drank to forget his painful memories.

But somehow Ed made it back. He made it back to his family, to the land of the Fort Albany First Nation, located on the southern shore of the mighty Albany where it meets James Bay. Ed turned to ceremony, to his elders, and to old teachings to find his way back to the land and to himself.

And that is why we are cruising down the Albany River on a freezing day in July. Inside the small cabin, nearly a dozen teens from Fort Albany First Nation are huddled together for warmth around a kitchen table. The tall, gawky youths — almost all dressed in various shades of black and with ball caps on — may have been born and bred in Fort Albany, but this is their very first trip out into the land to learn traditional ways of living, from skinning a fish to sleeping on the soft, mossy ground.

"When will Little Brother finally stand up and say, 'Enough'?" Ed wonders, the rain using his long black-and-grey ponytail as a vessel to travel down to the small of his back and whoosh off him. He fears Little Brother has lost his way.

Just to the south, vast pit mines have laid waste to miles and miles of once pristine boreal forests. Known as the northern lungs of the Earth, the forests act as massive "carbon sinks," taking carbon dioxide out of the atmosphere.[3] They extend across the northern hemisphere, from Canada to Norway and Russia.

But now development encroaches on this land. Prospectors mine for precious diamonds hidden in deep pipes of rock or for traces of chromite, the mineral used to make stainless steel appliances. Every single day that it is in operation, the Victor Diamond Mine, owned by De Beers, one of the global gem giants, is permitted to pump between 79 million and 150 million litres of water from the Victor pit in order to access the diamond deposits. The excess water is then pumped into the Attawapiskat, a 748-kilometre-long river that runs south of the Albany. The displacement of all this water, Ed says, upsets the fragile ecosystems.[4]

The Cree have travelled these riverbanks, watched and protected the water and land surrounding it, for as long as they can remember. The Albany weaves like a thick snake, separating the resource-rich North from the hungry, ever-growing South, which is constantly demanding to be fed. Big Brother demands what Little Brother has in order to feed its industry, construct its sprawling urban housing developments, and manufacture goods for its consumer-driven society.

You see, notes Ed, the more we damage the Earth, the more our Indigenous selves will wither and hollow with the destruction of the land. Take the Indian out of the land, away from their language, culture, mode of thought, and traditional way of living, and you begin to destroy their soul. Each bulldozer ploughing through the muskeg is like another cut.

Ed tells me that some people have suffered so much they disappear into the bush and never come back. This act is symbolic of taking one's life. It disrupts the rhythm of life, because everyone born on Turtle Island has their path set for them, he says, and the choice to end your life is not yours to make — it is the Creator's.

And this is why he piles teenagers onto his raft, along with his younger brother Mike Metatawabin, a former deputy grand chief of Nishnawbe Aski Nation. Like his older brother Ed, Mike is a survivor of St. Anne's. Since he was five years old, he has been carrying the memory of his time there in a nightmare he can't forget. In the dream he is in a church with all the other boys from school. When he looks up, instead of seeing Jesus, he sees the Devil himself nailed to the crucifix.

"That nightmare traumatized me, and I couldn't tell anyone," Mike says. "I kept asking myself, 'What did I do? What sin did I commit? Am I a bad boy?' I lived with this dream for decades."

Ed and Mike have watched many of their generation fall victim to the pain of the past — addictions, violence, suicide. They know too well those hollow feelings of being lost.

But the brothers have survived. They've made it through the unimaginable. They are still here.

And they know that to heal the spirits of the next generation, they must reintroduce the youth to who they are. Where they come from. Their true culture and rites of passage.

Elder Sam Achneepineskum and I often talk about these things, often in a Tim Hortons coffee shop as he sips his favourite vice — the triple-triple, a coffee with three sugars and triple cream.

Sam is a treasure from Ogoki Post, Marten Falls First Nation. He is a survivor of three residential schools. McIntosh Indian Residential School in Vermilion Bay, Northwestern Ontario, was his first stop. When the student residence at McIntosh burned down in 1965, he was sent to Cecilia Jeffrey Indian Residential School. There he joined his large extended family, including his cousin Chanie Wenjack, who at age twelve ran away from the school late one Sunday in October and tried to walk nearly a thousand kilometres home to Ogoki. Chanie's body was found on the railway tracks outside of Reddit, Ontario, where he had died of exposure. Frontman Gord Downie of the Canadian rock band the Tragically Hip was so haunted by Chanie's story that he memorialized the young boy's life in a book called *Secret Path*, and then an album and concert tour. Chanie's story has come to symbolize the stories of the 150,000 children who were sent to residential school.

Sam's last residential school was the notorious

St. Anne's in Fort Albany, where Ed Metatawabin and his brother Mike were sent.

Every time I am in Thunder Bay, my mother's home territory, I call up Sam. He has become an Elder not just to me but to all of Nishnawbe Aski Nation. He is the keeper of language and of stories, the holder of ceremonies and of hands for those who need him. And he doles out his wisdom for the small price of a large Tim Hortons triple-triple.

On this cold April morning, Sam and I are sitting in my rental car outside the Airlane, a 1950s-era motor hotel across the street from the airport on the outskirts of town. My Aunt Connie used to work there, back in the day when the Airlane was the place to be. On this particular morning, which is grey and threatens snow, Sam is telling me the story of how four events forever changed our people's relationship with the land, a story he heard from Louis Bird, a Cree Elder from Weenusk First Nation, also known as Peawanuck, near the southern shores of Hudson Bay.

"The first group of people to arrive here were the fur traders. They changed our relationship with the land, and we took more than was needed," he says, sipping his coffee. "Now we were doing something we never did before: we were competing to get more than anyone else. Before, we only hunted what we needed. When we had more, we would share with others, because we believed if we shared, we would be blessed with abundance." Inside the hotel, a Secret Path education conference is taking place. Members of the community have come together to figure out how the story of Chanie Wenjack can be incorporated into the Ontario elementary school curriculum. Sam's cousin and Chanie's sister, Daisy Munroe, a school principal, is in attendance along with her daughter Harriet Visitor, a teacher.

"Secondly, the missionaries came along and they changed our relationship with the Creator, with God," Sam says. "They brought the Bible and imposed their beliefs and their understanding of God. It changed our understanding of God, our relationship with the Creator. Before they came, our people believed in one way. If you add more ways, belief becomes diluted and weak."

The churches convinced the government that they couldn't do their missionary work properly because the people were scattered throughout the land, Sam says. "Then the Indian Act was put in place, and it took people off the land and forced them on reserves. Then came the residential schools, which removed the children from their families,

their communities, and the land. They got disconnected from everything. Knowledge was not passed
down. Parents lost their purpose, their whole reason for being. And this is where we are today."

IN 1493, ONE YEAR after Christopher Columbus
landed on the shores of the Americas, Pope
Alexander VI of the Roman Catholic Church created a series of orders called papal bulls, which
were used to legitimize the Spanish Empire's con-
quest of the Americas. These orders, now known
as the Doctrine of Discovery, are based on the concept of *terra nullius*, Latin for "land belonging to
no one."[5]

The phrase is interesting—"land belonging to no
one." In and of itself, it can be interpreted in many
ways. For First Peoples, that the land belongs to no
one means the land belongs to everyone. Within
this context, land cannot be owned; land is a common holding. This understanding derives from the
Indigenous peoples' traditional way of living, from
the Plains Indians in North America, tracking the
buffalo for the hunt, to the Sami in Scandinavia,
herding the reindeer while following their natural
migration patterns, to the Inuit of northern Canada

and Greenland, crossing the land and frozen sea by dogsled to hunt the seal and the whale. Human life adapts to the laws of nature; the natural world does not adapt to human life. The Indigenous peoples view their relationship to the land, to the water, to all life on Earth, as sacred; separation from the land is equivalent to a spiritual separation.[6]

For the Roman Catholic Church and the competing Spanish, Portuguese, Dutch, British, and French empires, that the land belonged to no one applied to the rules of territorial acquisition and occupation formulated during this age of "discovery." This interpretation did two seemingly contradictory things. First, within the context of empire building, it nullified the physical existence of the First Peoples, who did not factor into the global political order. By contrast, within the context of the Church, it acknowledged the presence of Indigenous Nations whose populations could help bolster Christianity's dominance among the major world religions. The papal bulls ordered that "the Catholic faith and the Christian religion be exalted and be everywhere increased and spread, that the health of souls be cared for and that barbarous nations be overthrown and brought to the faith itself."[7] The Doctrine of Discovery was born as a pact between church and state, one that would evolve to have tremendous implications for Indigenous Nations.

From the eighteenth to the twentieth centuries, as the age of empire waned, the new emerging nation-states continued to exercise the latter interpretation of the Doctrine of Discovery.[8] On July 4, 1776, one year into the American Revolutionary War, the Thirteen Colonies declared independence from Great Britain, thus forming the United States of America. Following the end of the war in 1783, the British Empire and the United States signed the Treaty of Paris, which recognized the U.S. as an independent republic. No provisions were made for the sovereignty of the Native American Nations. Land promised to those who had fought alongside the British army was ceded to the Americans, who saw the Ohio Country, western New York, Pennsylvania, Virginia, and Kentucky as theirs.[9] The Native Americans, who had been warring with the colonial powers since the sixteenth century, would continue to battle for their existence.

In North America, territorial acquisition and occupation was legalized through treaties with separate Indigenous Nations; the amassment of Christian converts was executed through the establishment of church-run residential schools.

Between 1778 and 1871, the U.S. Congress ratified 371 treaties or legally binding agreements that established the recognition of hundreds of American Indian Nations, legally constituted reservation land, and outlined the rights and responsibilities of both parties.[10] By making hundreds of separate land deals with individual American Indian Nations or small coalitions and confederacies, the U.S. government set up a tactical divide-and-conquer strategy in its quest to forge the new republic.[11]

As the nation continued to expand, the terms of the treaties went unfulfilled and wars broke out. On May 28, 1830, President Andrew Jackson signed the Indian Removal Act, which legally entitled the president to resettle all American Indians who lived east of the Mississippi River. Before he became president, Jackson had solidified his reputation as a military leader who fought for the settlers of the west during the 1813–14 Creek War. The Creek War began as a civil war among the Muscogee, or Creek Indians, over the degree to which they should adopt American ways of life.[12] Then the United States got involved in the conflict and waged war against the Red Sticks, a traditionalist faction of the Muscogee. The year-long battle was so brutal that Jackson himself admitted in a letter to his wife that "the carnage was dreadful."[13] By the end, the Muscogee Nation was shattered; the terms of the Treaty of Fort Jackson granted the United States half of their territory — twenty million acres of land, accounting for half of Alabama and parts of southern Georgia.[14]

While some Native Americans agreed to resettlement, the Cherokee — who had faced expulsion from Georgia after the discovery of gold in 1829, and ongoing pressure from settlers who wanted to establish cotton plantations on the fertile land — would not yield to the terms of the Indian Removal Act. But by 1838, those who resisted were forcibly removed from their homes and sent out west, or they were held in prison camps. Four thousand Cherokee died from disease, exposure, or starvation in a historical event now known as the Trail of Tears.[15]

During the American Civil War (1861–65), U.S. general William Tecumseh Sherman famously said, "We have made more than one thousand treaties with various Indian tribes, and have not kept one of them."[16] The irony is not lost on us that the general was named after Tecumseh, the great Shawnee chief who formed a confederacy of Native American

Nations to fight the U.S. alongside Britain during the War of 1812. Sherman was also responsible for clearing the Plains Indians in order to make way for the railroads and the telegraph. In 1862, miners struck gold, precipitating a rush of settlers on the traditional hunting grounds of the Sioux, Kiowa, and Comanche Nations, who again resisted expulsion from their lands.[17] By the late 1860s and into the 1870s, Sherman had ordered the slaughter of five million bison.[18] The destruction of the buffalo meant the destruction of the Plains Indians — the loss of their food source, their hunting grounds, and ultimately their entire way of life would sever their attachment to the land in this violent act of cultural cleansing. One colonel was heard saying, "Kill every buffalo you can! Every buffalo dead is an Indian gone."[19]

Between 1540 and 1924, the Nations battled first the British and the colonists and then the United States and the settlers in what historians call the American Indian Wars. For nearly four centuries, the Indigenous peoples of this land have fought the hegemonic powers.

One of the most famous acts of resistance was led by Chief Joseph of the Nez Percé Nation, whose homeland was the Wallowa Valley in Oregon. In

1860, thousands of miners descended upon the region, following the discovery, again, of gold. The Nez Percé were offered a treaty in which their five thousand square miles of land would be reduced to five or six hundred. The government called it the Lapwai Treaty, but many of the Nez Percé referred to it as the "thief treaty."[20] In 1873, President Ulysses S. Grant signed a new federal order allotting the Wallowa Valley to the Nez Percé. Two years later, the federal government reversed its decision. In 1877, Chief Joseph led seven hundred Nez Percé (fewer than two hundred of whom were warriors) on a 1,400-mile march to Canada, where he would seek political asylum for his people. Over a three-month period, the Nez Percé successfully fought four major battles and several small clashes against two thousand U.S. soldiers, until they were defeated just forty miles from the Canadian border at the Bears Paw Mountains in Montana.[21] The trek is considered one of the greatest military retreats in history, prompting even General William Tecumseh Sherman to acknowledge, "The Indians throughout displayed a courage and skill that elicited universal praise... [they] fought with almost scientific skill, using advance and rear guards, skirmish lines, and field fortifications."[22]

The press followed Chief Joseph's campaign closely, and he was deemed a war hero. General Nelson A. Miles, who finally halted the Nez Percé's exodus north, famously called him "the Napoleon of Indians," after the French emperor Napoleon Bonaparte, who is considered one of the world's greatest military leaders.[23]

Despite their defeat, Chief Joseph never stopped petitioning for the return of his people to the Wallowa Valley. In 1879, he went to Washington to meet with President Rutherford Hayes and, in a speech before diplomats and members of cabinet and Congress, chronicled the Nez Percé's history with the settlers: "We did not know there were other people besides the Indian until about one hundred winters ago, when some men with white faces came to our country. They brought many things with them to trade for furs and skins."[24]

Chief Joseph went on to describe how in 1805 his people had befriended two men, Captain Meriwether Lewis and Second Lieutenant William Clark. From May 1804 to September 1806, Lewis and Clark had been sent by President Thomas Jefferson on an expedition to find a route to the Pacific Ocean, thereby becoming the first Americans to explore the western frontier. Chief

Joseph noticed that Lewis and Clark had allowed their friends to build houses and farms on the land. At first the Nez Percé did not mind, because they had been treated well and thought they and the newcomers could live together. But over time the relationship changed:

> Year after year we have been threatened, but no war was made upon my people until General Howard came to our country two years ago and told us that he was the white war-chief of all that country. He said: "I have a great many soldiers at my back. I am going to bring them here, and then I will talk to you again. I will not let white men laugh at me the next time I come. The country belongs to the Government, and I intend to make you go upon the reservation."[25]

After meeting with President Hayes in 1879, Chief Joseph met with President William McKinley in 1897 and with President Theodore Roosevelt in 1903. He died on September 23, 1904, at the age of sixty-four. In his obituary, the *New York Times* wrote, "His death removes the most notable figure remaining among all the Indian tribes... He enjoyed the highest respect of all who knew him."[26]

THE 1800S WAS A CENTURY of massive expansion and land acquisition by the United States of America. By 1853, the nation had expanded with the Louisiana Purchase, which accounts for 23.3 percent of current U.S. territory; the acquisition of Texas and Florida from Spain; the expansion west into the Oregon Territory; and the cession of modern-day California, Nevada, Utah, and parts of Arizona, Colorado, and New Mexico, following the Mexican-American War.[27] In 1800, the Indigenous population, minus Hawaii and Alaska, was estimated to be around 600,000; by 1890, that number was reduced to 228,000.[28]

Beginning in 1879, the U.S. government introduced the American Indian boarding schools, or Indian Residential Schools, in order to assimilate what was left of the Indigenous population into the dominant society. The state-funded, church-run schools were modelled after the first off-reserve educational facility, the Carlisle Indian Industrial School in Carlisle, Pennsylvania, founded by Captain Richard Henry Pratt. Pratt believed Indians were born "blank," and that removal from their culture and traditional family structure would allow them to be modelled and shaped into Americans.

"A great general has said that the only good Indian is a dead one, and that high sanction of his destruction has been an enormous factor in promoting Indian massacres," Pratt said. "In a sense, I agree with the sentiment, but only in this: that all the Indian there is in the race should be dead. Kill the Indian in him, and save the man."[29]

Indigenous children as young as six years old were removed from their reservations and taken away from their families. At school, their hair was shorn, their names were changed, and they were forbidden from speaking their original languages.[30] By 1900, 150 schools had been set up across the country.

In Canada, it was Duncan Campbell Scott, superintendent of the Department of Indian Affairs from 1913 to 1932, who was the chief architect of the Government of Canada's notorious Indian Residential School system.

Scott first became engrossed with the "Indian problem" in 1895, when he was acting superintendent general of Indian Affairs. At that time, he requested that the minister of justice authorize the forced removal of every Indigenous child from their family so they could be sent to residential school.[31]

Over the summers of 1905 and 1906, Scott was one of three treaty commissioners sent by the Dominion of Canada and the Province of Ontario to negotiate the terms of Treaty No. 9, one of eleven numbered land-rights treaties the Government of Canada signed with First Nations. The land in question now encompasses 338,000 square kilometres between the Great Lakes and James Bay, an area roughly the size of France, and is the traditional territory of the Ojibwe, Cree, and Oji-Cree peoples.

Scott, along with treaty commissioners Samuel Stewart and Daniel G. MacMartin, who was the province's representative, journeyed north by canoe to meet with the First Nations and convince them to sign over their land to the Crown. In a letter dated November 6, 1905, to the superintendent of Indian Affairs, Scott outlines in great detail his portage travels by canoe throughout Northern Ontario in the pursuit of a 233,000-square-kilometre tract of "provincial lands drained by the Albany and the Moose River systems," to "admit to treaty any Indian whose hunting grounds cover portions of the Northwest Territories lying between the Albany river, the district of Keewatin and Hudson bay, and to set aside reserves in that territory."[32]

The party left Dinorwic, Ontario, at the end of June 1905, travelled up to Osnaburgh, which is now Mishkeegogamang First Nation, and continued along to Lake St. Joseph, the start of the Albany

River basin. They made stops at First Nations along their journey, including Lac Seul, where they made "an attempt to discourage the dances and medicine feasts" taking place on the reserve.[33]

Scott's letter describes exactly which route they took and notes that communities often had a large Anglican or Roman Catholic church. He remarks upon the influence of the clergy — from Moose Factory to Fort Albany to Fort Hope — who acted as translators for the Ojibwe and Cree. The sway of religious leaders at this time cannot be overstated. In some communities, it is still strong to this day.

Some communities had both a church and a Hudson's Bay Company trading post, where animal furs were traded for goods such as sugar, flour, and kettles. For centuries the Ojibwe and Cree in the North had traded with the Hudson's Bay Company. Their relationship with the company was based on treaties, which were seen as sacred. According to documents from the Lake Superior fur trade, the Ojibwe and Cree had expected to receive help from their trading partners if ever they were in need. They would refer to a trader as *ogimaa*, which means "leader" in Ojibwe, but this person was not their boss; he was the one who had responsibility for the people. In Ojibwe and Cree culture, leadership didn't mean power; it meant caring. After two centuries of fur trading, they expected that the Crown, too, would protect and help the Indigenous people in times of need.[34] But it would take decades for First Nations to fully understand that the Crown had no such intention and that they would be betrayed.

By the late nineteenth century, the HBC compacts had diminished. In 1884, Chief Louis Espagnol, from the Robinson-Superior Treaty area, around Lake Superior, said, "The construction of the Canadian Pacific Railway has opened up the country in the neighbourhood of Lake Pogamasing to White Trappers who deprive the Indians of the Beaver (which they carefully preserved, never taking all, but leaving some to increase) and as the Whites kill and destroy all they can, the consequence will be that no Beaver will be left in that section of country."[35]

By the time the treaty commissioners arrived in some parts of Northern Ontario, the people of the upper Albany River and from the headwaters of the Missinaibi and Abitibi Rivers were all suffering — the fur trade was collapsing.[36] The area was also recovering from years of harsh weather, and many had suffered from a measles outbreak. As the commissioners travelled farther north into the hinterland, the First Nations people looked increasingly hungry and unwell.

In exchange for a huge swath of land rich in natural resources such as gold, lumber, and hydroelectric power from the river systems, the signatories of Treaty No. 9 were to receive four dollars a year — one dollar less than what the Treaty No. 3 Indians were receiving — and the commissioners said they would work together with the First Nations to find them a suitable place for their reserves.[37] The Indians understood that this would be territory they could use on their own, away from white men, and that they were free to hunt and fish and roam the land as always.

"When it was explained to them that they could hunt and fish as of old and they were not restricted as to territory, the Reserve merely being a home for them where no white man could interfere or trespass upon, that the land was theirs for ever, they gladly accepted the situation," MacMartin wrote in his recently discovered diary.[38]

Read the fine print of Treaty No. 9 and it says something quite different. Economic progress, business, and settlement would take precedence over any Indigenous hunting, fishing, or land rights. The state's objective was simple: to get the First Nations to "cede, release, surrender and yield" their land to the Crown.[39] In his diary, MacMartin corroborates the Indigenous peoples' claim that the commissioners misrepresented the terms of the treaty that appeared in the final written agreement.[40] In 2013, a lawsuit launched by late Grand Chief Stan Louttit of the Mushkegowuk Council claimed that the Canadian and Ontario governments did not keep their oral promises to the Indigenous people and that they failed to properly explain the terms of the treaty. The council argues that the government has "no power or right under Treaty 9 to unilaterally restrict or extinguish" the Mushkegowuk people's rights by allowing resource companies to develop on their land.[41]

In effect, the First Nations lost the land that they and their ancestors had always walked on — for four dollars a year, a sum that has never been adjusted for inflation.

One must assume the chiefs took the document in good faith. They believed the treaty process was cementing a reciprocal relationship, one they undertook to gain agricultural and economic help in times of hardship, famine, and transition. It was seen as a mutual agreement of respect. As scholar John Long noted in *Treaty No. 9: Making the Agreement to Share the Land in Far Northern Ontario in 1905*, we must now "read between the lines (or 'beyond the words') to ensure we understand the very different world views involved."[42]

Significantly, all those who signed the treaty were told that their children would be given a proper Canadian education at a residential school. Indigenous culture was considered inferior and seen as savagery. Christian missionaries who administered Canada's residential school system (paid for by the federal government) also led campaigns to ban traditional practices such as the Potlatch, the Sun Dance, and marriage ceremonies. The churches sought government support for their missionary work. They wanted to turn the Indians into good Christians and farmers, believing this would lead them to salvation, and the federal government wanted them assimilated into Canadian society so it would no longer have any fiduciary responsibility towards them.[43]

Finally, in 1920, when Duncan Campbell Scott was at the height of his career as superintendent of Indian Affairs, he amended the Indian Act to include the mandatory enrolment in residential school of Indigenous children between the ages of seven and fifteen.[44]

First introduced in 1876, nine years after Canadian Confederation, the Indian Act is a federal statute that governs every aspect of an Indigenous person's life, from land management to education to cultural ceremony and even status and identity. It is a registry of all First Nations people in Canada. Those who have proven status — based on the Government of Canada's strict criteria — are given a ten-digit number signifying that they have been sanctioned as official Indians and are kept on a roll. The policy also kept First Nations on reserves allocated on Crown land and sanctioned the cruel removal of children from their families, their communities, to be sent to one of the 139 Indian Residential Schools across the country. The Indian Act has been described as a form of apartheid, controlling Indigenous people's lives to this very day.

In 1920, Scott famously told a parliamentary committee, "Our object is to continue until there is not a single Indian in Canada that has not been absorbed into the body politic."[45]

In this way, Scott successfully created, and helped to enforce, an oppressive system of segregation and assimilation. Nearly 150,000 First Nations, Métis, and Inuit children were sent to the residential schools. An estimated 6,000 Indigenous children died because they were being mistreated, abused, neglected, or starved, all under the pretense of receiving an education.[46]

THE GOVERNMENT OF CANADA'S acts of systemic segregation and racial discrimination extended to the Far North, past the Canadian provinces, where Inuit, a distinct people, have lived for thousands of years. This area is called Inuit Nunangat. *Nunangat* is the Inuktut word for the land, water, and ice that make up their traditional cultural space, which comprises 35 percent of Canada's land mass, including 50 percent of its coastline. The area is divided into the four regions Inuit have traditionally occupied: Inuvialuit (in the Northwest Territories), the territory of Nunavut, Nunavik (northern Quebec), and Nunatsiavut (northern Labrador).[47]

For generations, Inuit have lived by the seasons, which, depending on the region, are split into five or six distinct periods.[48] *Auyarq* is the summer of constant sun, when time seems endless and people travel on land and by sea. *Ukiaksaaq* is the waning days of autumn. *Ukiaq* is early winter, when the land begins to ice over. *Ukiuq* is mid-winter, when the days get progressively shorter and the nights longer. *Upingarqsaaq* is late winter, when the Arctic is submerged in twenty-four-hour darkness. And *Upingaaq* is spring, when the ice begins to melt and the sunlight makes its return.[49]

Inuit developed their traditional culture and lifestyle by adapting to these seasons and the Arctic climate. They used the animals' natural migration patterns as a guide by which they could hunt seal and whale. In Nunavut, the early spring is the time of the seal pups, the Arctic hare; it is a time of hunting and fishing. Later spring, around June, is the season of nesting geese, clams, the beluga whale and walrus hunts. In the summer, Inuit prepare the caribou skin, the Arctic char runs, and the berries can be picked. The fall is the time of the caribou hunt and the time to sew clothes for the coming winter. The winter is the season of the denning polar bear.[50]

For thousands of years, Inuit have employed *qimmiit*, or sled dogs, to traverse the winter landscape. The dogs were integral to the Inuit's survival. Not only could they find their way

home in a minus-fifty-degree-Celsius snowstorm, they could sense where the ice was thin,
warning their owners of danger. They also helped
hunt polar bears and could sniff out the seals'
breathing holes in the ice. The teams of seven
or eight dogs that make up sled packs were part
of the family and treated as such. Neither could
survive without the other.[51]

The market demand for fur, popularized by
European fashion in the late nineteenth century,
had resulted in depletion of species in the south.[52]
Prior to the arrival of the HBC, Inuit and their ancestors had limited contact with Europeans. Sometime
between 1100 and 1300 AD, the Thule made contact
with the Vikings in Greenland, where they attacked
the Norse settlements. By the fifteenth century, the
Thule had overtaken the territory.[53] In 1575, the
English explorer Martin Frobisher journeyed to
Baffin Island in search of the Northwest Passage,
which would provide a quicker route to Asia. His
arrival marked the first time in the modern era that
someone of European descent had settled in the
Arctic for the winter season.[54] Thereafter, for hundreds of years, explorers came to the area looking
for the fabled passage to Asia. But the coming of
the mighty HBC would prove to be devastating for

Inuit in the Far North, just as it was for the First Nations and Métis in the south.

Families began to settle around the posts. Some engaged in the profitable fur trade, while others worked as labourers. The fur trade also brought missionaries and the Royal Canadian Mounted Police. With the influx of southerners, towns were constructed, and the Inuit lifestyle quickly shifted from living off the land, following the animals and the seasons, to a stationary urban existence. The Indian Residential School system was introduced to ensure the assimilation of the next genera-tion. Around the same time, the Cold War pushed Canada to assert its Arctic sovereignty to ward off jurisdictional claims by the Soviet Union and the United States. The government set up communi-ties such as Grise Fiord and constructed the DEW Line— the Distant Early Warning Line, a system of radar stations that would warn of a Soviet inva-sion by land, air, or sea.

Though Inuit were not under the jurisdiction of the Indian Act, the Government of Canada used the same tactics to quell the peoples of the North. In addition to relegating families to the towns and sending their kids to residential school, from the 1950s to the 1970s the RCMP culled the sled dogs, now confined to the towns with their owners. Thousands of dogs died of disease brought to the North by white settlers; the rest became targets of mass killings. Because at certain times of the year and also during certain stages of development the dogs were allowed to roam free, they were deemed a "law enforcement issue," threatening the safety of the settler population. Inuit Elders remember seeing the dogs shot and killed when they were harnessed up and ready to go. In some cases the police laughed in front of their owners. Dozens of dogs were piled into pyramids and their corpses were burned.[55]

Just as the massacre of the bison in nineteenth-century America helped usher in the demise of the Plains Indians' traditional way of life, so too was the killing of the dogs a powerful act of subjugation. Both acts symbolically severed the Indigenous peoples' spiritual connection to the land by eliminating a major source of their sustenance and economy. The words of Lieutenant Richard Henry Pratt, founder of the boarding schools for Indigenous children in America, apply equally to this practice: "Kill the Indian and save the man."

There are two different versions of what happened from 1950 to 1970. In 2005, the Government of Canada's House of Commons Standing Committee on Aboriginal Affairs and Northern Development first heard from witnesses of the killing of the dogs. It was noted that the dogs' deaths occurred around the time of Inuit resettlement. The committee ordered a public inquiry, but it was never sanctioned by the federal government. Instead, the government asked the RCMP to conduct a "comprehensive review" of what came to be known as the "dog slaughter."[56]

In 2006, the RCMP released a twenty-six-page report exonerating members of the force. It maintained that the killings were completely legal and were never part of a "conspiracy" with the explicit motive of forcing Inuit to stop hunting and live in permanent settlements. By contrast, Inuit saw the act as part of a "series of interconnected government policies and laws put into effect and enforced by the RCMP, which quickly undermined traditional Inuit ways of living."[57]

The conclusions of the report, and its assessment of how Inuit were treated over that twenty-year period, prompted the Qikiqtani Inuit Association, an organization that represents the people of Qikiqtani, or the Baffin Island area, to conduct its own, Inuit-led inquiry, called the Qikiqtani Truth

Commission. Taking issue with the RCMP report's apparent suggestion that the hundreds of Inuit witness testimonies were unreliable or incorrect, the QTC expanded the scope of its inquiry to include an examination of RCMP–Inuit relations.

The QTC pointed out that the RCMP had an elevated stature in the North because it not only acted as law enforcer but also, in the absence of any structured northern government, fulfilled the role of governance in the Baffin Island region. In the 1950s, RCMP–Inuit relations began to change when policies of assimilation were introduced and enforced. Children were taken from their homes and sent to residential school; churches were established; parents were forced to live in permanent communities. As military bases were set up in the region, about one hundred autonomous Inuit groups were moved into thirteen settlements. The RCMP was complicit in the forced relocation of the Inuit and the government's appropriation of their traditional lands. Around this time, the Canadian government revised the territory's Ordinance Respecting Dogs, which outlawed the traditional Inuit way of handling the animals.[58]

Kopa Mike remembers when the RCMP took their dogs away. "The police would shoot the dogs," she tells me, her hands folded in her lap. She recalls her husband telling her about witnessing it. "One day, the RCMP came and they started to beat the dogs. One dog went under the house and an officer shot it. The dog didn't have a chance."

Kopa is sitting in the Elder's Qammaq in downtown Iqaluit, the capital city of the territory of Nunavut. Located on the southern end of Baffin Island, Iqaluit (meaning "place of fish") has a population of about eight thousand. The Qammaq (Inuit for "sod hut") is a drop-in centre for Elders who want to socialize and get a hot lunch for two dollars. In late May, the city is still trying to thaw out, and the crisp Arctic air blows a fine dust that settles on your clothes and in your hair. In the 1940s, the U.S. military set up a base here and the residents were moved inland, first to Apex, just a few minutes along the coast, where the Hudson's Bay Company opened up a trading post in 1949.

Iqaluit is a city of contrasts. The buildings are brightly coloured; the fibreglass schools look like blue-and-white Lego spaceships. The Anglican church, St. Jude's Cathedral, is shaped like a giant white igloo. Construction materials have to be able to withstand the long, harsh winters, and they need to be easily transportable, because the weather makes consistent year-round shipping impossible — air travel is the only way to reach this remote part of the country twelve months of the year. Iqaluit runs on diesel, which is brought up in bulk during the summer months and stored beside the dump. In May 2014, the dump caught fire, creating a massive plume of smoke that could be seen throughout town. The fire, dubbed "dumpcano," burned for months on end. The busiest intersection in town, which everyone calls "the four corners," is a four-way stop with a Royal Bank, government buildings, and tourist shops selling Inuit art and sculptures. There are no traffic lights in Iqaluit, just stop signs. The new beer and wine store opened in September 2017, and it always seems to have a lineup to get in. The city has a large, modern hospital, but it does not have a mental health or addictions treatment centre.

Iqaluit is split up into neighbourhoods including Happy Valley and Tundra Valley. One of the main roads is called the "Road to Nowhere," and it is — it leads right out of town and straight to a shooting range on the tundra.

There is a severe housing shortage. Those with government jobs often have access to reserved housing, but for everyone else, trying to find a place to live is extremely difficult. Large extended families often share a one- or two-bedroom apartment, and family members have to sleep in shifts. About 52 percent reside in homes that are overcrowded by federal standards. The housing shortage leads to high rents, and demand is constant because of the Inuit's high birth rate — about 33 percent of the population is aged zero to fourteen, and 34 percent is aged fifteen to thirty-four; the median age is twenty-three. The median income is $23,485, and only 47.5 percent of those of working age are employed.[59]

Kopa was born in Cape Dorset (or Kinngait in Inktitut), on the southern tip of Baffin Island, in 1951, a time of great change in the North. Inuit always called this region Sikusiilaq, but in 1631 the British renamed it after the fourth Earl of Dorset, Edward Sackville.

Kopa's parents were fierce hunters, and she and her six siblings lived traditionally. In 1956, Inuit were being urged to move to one of the permanent settlements, so her parents gathered up her and her siblings and they travelled by dogsled to what is now Iqaluit. Her parents were told that Kopa and her siblings had to go to school, and if her parents didn't voluntarily send the children to residential school, the police would. They were also warned that they would lose their child tax credit (or "baby bonus"), a monthly sum that helped pay some expenses. She remembers the police coming into their camps and threatening to take the kids away. In the mid-1960s, she was enrolled in the Churchill Vocational Centre on the Hudson Bay coast and stayed for just one year before she became pregnant with her first child at the age of fourteen. Kopa wanted to go back to school, but her boy-friend wanted her to stay at home and take care of their family.

Kopa saw her people experience a massive cul-tural shift as they adapted to the confines of urban life. And once the dogs were gone, the people were no longer able to travel the great distances to visit relatives and friends or to hunt.

"Everywhere, the dogs died," Kopa says. The RCMP would shoot the dogs on the ice, then burn them. When the ice melted, the bodies sank into the water.

The absence of freedom changed everything, she says. The people were suddenly overcome by a listlessness, an existential and spiritual emptiness.

Kopa had seven children; only four are still alive. Three of her sons died by suicide; her youngest son was only fifteen years old when he took his own life. She blames the scourges of alcohol and drugs, substances that numb people to their present circumstances and fuel the violence, the fights, the thievery. And she laments the loss of language among today's Inuit youth.

"When white people got control of the Inuit, it got worse," she says with a deep sigh, as the twenty-four-hour sun bleaches the curtains. "They can't control what they don't know."

THE POLICY OF EXTERMINATION, isolation, and assimilation repeats itself in the history of Indigenous Nations throughout the world, and still continues today. One of the most tragic examples is that of the Indigenous peoples of Brazil.

In 1969, Norman Lewis, an English travel writer and a journalist for the *Sunday Times*, published a shocking in-depth report titled "Genocide," which chronicled the near extinction of many of the Indigenous Nations in Brazil during the 1950s and 1960s.

The Portuguese colony wasn't established until 1549, more than fifty years after Christopher Columbus landed in the Caribbean, when Tomé de Sousa was sent over to become the governor general of the colony of Brazil. At the time, the Portuguese wanted to ward off threats from the surrounding Spanish colonies. In 1494, the Spanish and Portuguese had signed the Treaty of Tordesillas to divide the lands outside Europe between the two empires. They drew a line from pole to pole, about 370 leagues west of Cape Verde Island. All lands west would go to the Spanish Empire, and all lands east would go to the Portuguese.[60]

In 1500, King John II sent the minor nobleman Pedro Álvares Cabral with a large expeditionary force to India. The expedition veered off course in the Atlantic as they tried to catch winds to southern Africa. In April 1500, they spotted what they thought was an island, but it was in fact the South American mainland.[61]

On board was Pêro Vaz de Caminha, who wrote a detailed account of the expedition's landing. Caminha's first impressions of the Indigenous peoples they encountered inspired the French Enlightenment philosopher Voltaire to form his theory of the "noble savage."[62]

"They seem to be such innocent people that, if we could understand their speech and they ours, they would immediately become Christians, seeing that, by all appearances, they do not understand about any faith," Caminha wrote. "These people are good and have a fine simplicity. Any stamp we wish may be easily printed on them, for the Lord has given them good bodies and good faces, like good men."[63]

At the time, the Portuguese didn't fully appreciate this newly discovered land — nor the people they encountered. They noted that there were no cattle, goats, or sheep, and that the staple of the Indigenous diet was the hearty root vegetable cassava. There was no evidence of coveted minerals such as gold or diamonds, nor did they find any cities. In early May 1500, they loaded up their ships with water, and part of the expedition continued on to search for India, while another ship headed back to Portugal with a letter to the king from Caminha.[64]

Sousa arrived with 1,200 men and women — settlers, soldiers, and six young priests from the Society of Jesus, or Jesuits. A dozen captaincies were set up along the coast.[65] The colony, along with the Caribbean islands, was developed as a plantation economy for the Spanish and Portuguese empires. In Brazil, the major commodity was sugar cane. These plantations were run on Indigenous and African slave labour.

Norman Lewis marks this as the beginning of a long history of savage brutality against the original inhabitants of Brazil:

> Economic forces the newcomers could have never understood were about to transform them into slavers and assassins. The natives gave gracefully, and the invaders took what they offered with grasping hand, and when there was nothing left to give the enslavement and the murder began. The American continent was about to be overwhelmed by what [the French anthropologist and ethnologist] Claude Lévi-Strauss described 400 years later as "that monstrous and incomprehensible cataclysm which the development of Western civilisation was for so large and innocent a part of humanity."[66]

The Indigenous peoples were wiped out by epidemics of tuberculosis, measles, and influenza and suffered from venereal disease and eye ailments, not to mention wholesale torture and extermination by "mass burnings, the flayings, the disembowellings, and the mutilations." Those who managed to escape enslavement on the plantations were often under the rule of the Jesuits on their reservations, which Lewis likens to "religious concentration camps." Accounts of early European explorers suggest that the land was populous when they first arrived; historians estimate that the number of Indigenous people in South America was between three and six million. By the beginning of the twentieth century, it's estimated, that population had been reduced to about one million.[67]

But the main subject of Lewis's account was revelation of the genocide of the Indigenous peoples of Brazil in the 1950s and 1960s, first instigated by a boom in rubber. The demand for the commodity in world markets sparked a major land grab to establish plantations, resulting in extermination and enslavement of the Indigenous peoples. These atrocities were carried out with the implicit agreement, or even co-operation, of corrupt politicians and bureaucrats within the government's Indian Protection Service.[68]

The genocide was reminiscent of the early settlers and the establishment of the sugar cane plantations. Indigenous men, women, and children were tortured, raped, and slaughtered. Lewis vividly describes one episode involving the Cintas Largas, who lived in the upper reaches of the Aripuanã River in the Mato Grosso and Amazonas states in northwestern Brazil. When the legislative assembly of Mato Grosso took over the management of land ownership and sale from the federal government, it triggered a power struggle between the rubber tappers and the mineral prospectors, who were competing for valuable land. Under the leadership of Francisco de Brito — the general manager of the rubber firm Arruda and Junqueira of Juina-Mirim, and a notorious sadist — a group of rubber tappers was sent to clear an area near the upper reaches of the Aripuanã. They loaded a Cessna light plane with dynamite, which was dropped on a village that was preparing for Quarup, an annual one- to two-day traditional feast in which family members gather to honour their ancestors.

When the survivors of the attack were seen building a new settlement far up the Aripuanã, a group led by one of Brito's men, named Chico, made its way up the river and hacked through the forest to finish the job. One of the men in Chico's group described in horrifying detail the killing of the men, women, and children with Tommy guns and machetes. The village was burned and the bodies were thrown in the river. Episodes such as this were not uncommon.

Indigenous people in Brazil are still under attack

today. In the northwestern region of the country, the Guarani people survive daily threats of violence, persecution, political assassination, and forced removal from the land.

The biggest Guarani community is the Kaiowá, or "people of the forest." They are a spiritual people who for thousands of years have been on a relentless search for the "land without evil," a place where their ancestors said they could live eternally without pain or suffering.[69] It has been a near fruitless search. Following the arrival of the Portuguese, the Guarani's existence has been plagued by virus and disease, enslavement and massacres.

In the past century there has been massive deforestation of the Amazon rainforests for biofuel, soya and coffee plantations, mineral extraction, and cattle ranches. The Guarani, who once spread over 350,000 kilometres of their state, Mato Grosso do Sul (formed when Mato Grosso was divided in the 1970s), now live on tiny government-appointed reserves. On the Dourados reserve, twelve thousand Indigenous people populate a three-thousand-hectare plot of land.[70]

In November 2007, there seemed to be a government turnaround concerning Indigenous land rights. The Fundação Nacional do Índio, Brazil's

Indigenous affairs agency, along with the Ministry of Justice, the Public Prosecutor's Office, and twenty-three Indigenous leaders, signed the Termo de Ajustamento de Conduta, which stated that the government would identify thirty-six Guarani lands and demarcate seven large territories encompassing them. Those territories were supposed to return to Indigenous communities in April 2010.[71]

But that hasn't happened. The Guarani have not been welcomed back to their ancestral land. Instead, they have been met with court challenges, armed resistance, and brutal violence. According to the Missionary Council for Indigenous Peoples, forty-one Indigenous people were murdered in Mato Grosso do Sul in 2014.[72] In many circumstances, people have been forced to live in gutters on the side of the road, their personal belongings strung up between the trees.[73]

What is happening to the Indigenous people in Brazil is no less than a human rights emergency. What was and is transpiring is in violation of international laws and conventions, notwithstanding Brazil's own constitution, Article 231 of which states that "Indians shall have their social organization, customs, languages, creed and traditions recognized, as well as their original rights to the lands they traditionally occupy, it being incumbent upon the Union to demarcate them, protect and ensure respect for all their property."[74]

On August 29, 2015, twenty-four-year-old Guarani leader Semião Vilhalva was shot in the face on a dusty road in his own territory. He was looking for his young son.[75] Images captured shortly after his death show him face down on the ground, blood streaming from his head. The attack on Vilhalva came just one week after he and members of the Guarani community occupied a part of their ancestral lands. They now accuse the ranchers of hiring gunmen and claim that the shooting occurred with government agents in attendance.[76]

Vilhalva is the third Indigenous leader to be murdered in Mato Grosso do Sul in the past several years. Marcos Verón died in 2003 after he led a group in a *retomada*, or a retaking, of the Takuará's ancestral land. He was shot and beaten to death. No one has been charged with his murder. Nizio Gomes was killed in November 2011, while he was in the *retomada* camp. His body has never been found.[77]

In the wake of Vilhalva's murder, Guarani Elder Tonico Benites told the BBC, "This is a deliberate policy of genocide. It's a long legal process designed to kill our people, slowly but surely. Our rights are being violated and we don't have even the basic conditions to survive. So we have no choice but to occupy, to retake our lands — otherwise we can't survive as a people."[78]

In 2005, the Brazilian president, Luiz Inácio Lula da Silva, ratified an agreement to return a large parcel of Ñanderu Marangatú land back to the Guarani people; ratification is the last step before land recognition.[79] But the land was never returned to the Guarani. The ranchers petitioned the Supreme Court, and that same year they won, effectively stopping the land transfer. On December 15, armed gunmen, aided by Brazilian military personnel, evicted the Guarani.

In a report prepared for the United Nations by the human rights group Survival International, one survivor described the eviction:

> Helicopters flew very low over the area. Children were screaming and crying. Three people fainted and were taken to hospital. Everyone was crying and standing on the side of the road with nothing in the baking sun. We had nothing to eat. When the police weren't there, the ranchers

burned all our food, our clothes and documents.
They burned fifteen houses. The only things we
have left are the clothes on our bodies.[80]

For six months, the Ñanderu Marangatú community lived along the roadsides before they were
allowed to return to the 100 hectares of land that
was part of their territory agreement — a mere frac-
tion of the 9,300 hectares originally ordered.[81]

The Métis in Canada were also forced to live on
roadsides after the Northwest Rebellion in 1885.
The Métis, proud descendants of French fur traders and First Nations people, are a distinct nation
largely based in Western Canada, with their own
language, culture, music, dance, and flag. When
the Hudson's Bay Company handed Rupert's Land
over to the Canadian government, no provisions
were made for the Métis, who were living on the
land. Without land, the Métis were forced to live
along road allowances, on unused Crown land such
as hillsides, at the edges of First Nations reserves,
and on the outskirts of town or in forests. They
became known as "squatting communities" or the
"Road Allowance People."[82] Still today, the Métis
are denied rights as Status Indians and they have
been denied their own land or territory.

As a result of the murders of their Indigenous leaders, the state of their living conditions, and their near enslavement on plantations and ranches, Guarani youth suffer from substance-abuse issues and overrepresentation in prisons, and their suicide rate is among the highest in South America.

Marcos Homero Ferreira Lima, a Brazilian official in the public prosecutor's office in Dourados, Mato Grosso do Sul, says the situation requires urgent action:

> It is not an exaggeration to speak of genocide, since the series of events and actions committed against this group since the end of the 1990s has contributed to subjecting its members to conditions preventing their physical, cultural and spiritual existence. Children, young people, adults and the elderly are subjected to degrading experiences which directly harm their human dignity.[83]

On November 5, 2015, Amnesty International wrote an open letter to Brazil's president, Dilma Rousseff: "It is essential that the Indigenous Guarani-Kaiowá peoples have their land demarcated and delivered to them, so that they can engage in their livelihoods and spiritual and cultural practices in dignity."[84] The letter notes that the suicide rate for the Guarani-Kaiowá people is thirty-four times higher than that of the non-Indigenous population. Since 2007, Brazil's Special Secretariat for Indigenous Health reports, 351 Indigenous people have died by suicide.[85] Between 2011 and 2015, 44.8 percent of the suicides were carried out by children between the ages of ten and nineteen. And for every 100,000 suicide deaths, 15.2 are Indigenous.[86]

Rosalino Ortiz's nine-year-old daughter, Luciane, hung herself inside their thatched hut. Her mother said the children are dying by suicide because they have no land. "We don't have space anymore. In the old days we were free; now we are no longer free," she says. "So our young people look around them and think there is nothing left and wonder how they can live. They lose themselves and then they commit suicide."[87]

Some of the Indigenous Nations have pushed back. In December 2006, twenty-nine miners were killed for working without permission at a mine on the Cintas Largas reserve. The Cintas Largas leaders had been urged to take a stand by women who said the miners were raping girls as young as fourteen and bringing drugs into the community. The Cintas Largas had already seen thousands of their people massacred since the 1960s by miners and land speculators.[88] One chief interviewed by Larry Rohter, the South American bureau chief for the *New York Times* from 1999 to 2007, suddenly turned to the journalist and asked: "Why are your people so warlike?"[89]

Still the atrocities continue. As recently as September 2017, ten members of an uncontacted Indigenous tribe in the Amazon were murdered by gold miners while they were gathering eggs by the river. The gold miners bragged about the killings in a bar, where they showed off a hand-carved paddle they had taken from one of the victims.[90]

In July 2018, video footage of an uncontacted Indigenous man in the Amazon made international headlines. Known as the "Indigenous man in the hole," he was believed to be the lone survivor of a group of six who were attacked by farmers in 1995. He had been living by himself in the forest for twenty-two years.

"I understand his decision," said Altair Algayer, a regional coordinator for the Fundação Nacional do Índio in the state of Rondônia. "It is his sign of resistance, and a little repudiation, hate, knowing the story he went through."

"The fact he is still alive gives you hope," said Fiona Watson, the research and advocacy director of Survival International. "He is the ultimate symbol, if you like."[91]

THREE

THE THIRD SPACE

BEFORE AN ANISHINAABE WOMAN gives birth to a child, Elder Sam Achneepineskum tells me, she sings to them. She speaks to them when she is in a good place, and she thanks them for coming into the family's life.

The baby is also told stories of their history, so they know who they are when they are born; they are prepared. When they come screaming into being, they are met by a bevy of women, each of whom has a special role to play in the birthing process. Traditionally, when a child is born, the Elders come to give the child the name they will carry for the rest of their days. A naming ceremony can happen at any time. When it does, the child enters into the realm of the tribe.

Directly after birth, the placenta is planted firmly in the earth. The umbilical cord is also saved and buried to ensure the child's future connection with the land.

For one year, the child is not to touch the ground. A baby is carried in their mother's tiki-nagan, a wooden board outfitted with hides and furs that holds the baby snug until that special day when they are ready to walk on their own. When that day comes, the baby has a "Walking Out" ceremony, wherein they take their first step, feel the ground firmly beneath their feet. And then that child is one with the Earth.

These ceremonies are the beginnings of the rites of passage, the path to adulthood. If a child misses a stage, they become disconnected from who they are and where they come from. This is how an Anishinaabe child learns *Mino Bimaadiziwin*, or "leading a good life." One can choose to be Anishinaabe, to live the good life, to live the way one's ancestors wanted one to, but to do this one must return to the old teachings and learn to speak the language.[1] This is the way it is and the way it always will be.

Attachments, kinship, and family tell us who we are and where we come from. They give us a sense of dignity, a sense of belonging, right from birth. In Indigenous cultures, family units go beyond the traditional nuclear family living together in one house. Families are extensive networks of strong, connective kinship; they are often entire communities. If a child is orphaned or if their biological parents are unable to care for them, the broader family takes over the primary rearing of that child. Instead of having one mother, the child could have a number of maternal figures. But if a child is taken away from their parents, their extended family, their community, they suffer multiple losses.

Helen Milroy explained the concept of Australian Aboriginal kinship to me in a seventh-floor breakfast room in a modern hotel in downtown Stockholm. We were there to attend an International Initiative for Mental Health Leadership conference. The IIMHL is a collective of 3,500 mental health professionals from around the world. Member countries include Canada, the United States, Australia, New Zealand, England, Scotland, and Ireland. They meet annually to compare notes on best practices and the challenges they face in mental health.

Helen, a descendant of the Palyku people of the Pilbara region in Western Australia, is a maverick in her field. Born and raised in Perth, she grew up in an Aboriginal household, supported by her mother and grandmother, and went to medical school at the University of Western Australia. She worked at Princess Margaret Hospital, where she specialized in child sexual abuse. There she witnessed the failure of modern medicine to treat traumatized children. In response to her experience, she went back to school and became the first Aboriginal psychiatrist in Australia. Helen speaks with fierce moral authority arising from the collective wisdom of her life experience. For five years she was one of six commissioners on the Royal Commission into Institutional Responses to Child Sexual Abuse in Australia. Prompted by allegations against the Roman Catholic Church, the commission was established in 2013 to look into public and state institutions — schools, churches, sporting clubs, orphanages, disability services — and their responses to reports of child sexual abuse.

Helen travelled across the continent, interviewing nearly 2,000 of the 6,875 child sexual assault survivors.[2] More than 2,500 cases were referred back to authorities for investigation, and allegations were made against four thousand institutions all over Australia. However, by far the most allegations were made against the Catholic Church, where 4,400 children were said to have suffered sexual abuse.[3] Forty suicides were directly related to abuse by the Catholic clergy in the state of Victoria.[4] The Anglican Church received 1,115 abuse claims.[5]

In its final report, released in December 2017, the royal commission made more than four hundred recommendations, including setting up a national prevention strategy and a federal government Office for Child Safety.[6] The commission also created "A Brief Guide to the Final Report: Aboriginal and Torres Strait Island Communities," outlining key information as it pertained to Australia's First Peoples. Of the survivors the commission interviewed, 14.3 percent, or 985 people, identified as Aboriginal or Torres Strait Islander, two distinct Indigenous peoples.[7] The guide was put together to take into account the historical, social, cultural, and political factors that are unique to the Indigenous experience.

From 1910 to 1970, the Australian government forcibly removed Aboriginal and Torres Strait Islands children from their homes, separating them from their families. Many children were fostered out to or adopted by white families, while others were placed in orphanages or other government- or church-run institutions. It is estimated that fifty thousand children were victims of this policy, and they are now called the "Stolen Generations."[8]

The federal and state government policies were developed between 1869, with the establishment of the Victorian Central Board for the Protection of Aborigines, and 1969, with the abolishment of the New South Wales Aboriginal Welfare Board. These policies were influenced by theories of social Darwinism that portrayed Indigenous people as an inferior race. The goal was to eliminate the Aboriginal and Torres Strait peoples: they would either die out naturally or be assimilated into white society. As a result, family structures, so precious in the cultures, were completely dismantled and destroyed. Thousands upon thousands of children were adopted by white families or placed in institutions where they were physically and sexually abused and neglected, forced to reject their names and heritage, and told their parents were dead or didn't want them. They were given a substandard education, and when they left school they could do little else than become labourers or domestic workers. Their parents and grandparents were forced to live in poverty on missions, reserves, and stations, or "managed reserves," sanctioned under the paternalistic and controlling regulatory policies of the Aboriginal Protection Act, which is akin to the Indian Act in Canada.[9]

The government policies and procedures had a hugely detrimental effect on the life trajectories of Aboriginals and Torres Strait Islanders, acting like an invisible anchor around their necks. "The moments that should be shared and rejoiced by a family unit, for [my brother] and mum and I are forever lost. The stolen years that are worth more than any treasures are irrecoverable," said one survivor.[10]

These Indigenous peoples were largely jobless and lived in impoverished conditions in cities and small country towns; they fell into patterns of addiction and had poor health and lower life expectancies than the general population; they suffered from intense discrimination, both societal and systemic; and they became overrepresented in the prison system. Children routinely grew up with no sense of belonging, no sense of themselves or where they came from, so they began to do something that was largely unheard of before: they began to kill themselves. And so did their children and their grandchildren.

"When you are held as a child," Helen said over her coffee, "you look up and see yourself reflected in your mum's loving gaze. You feel loved, secure, and good. If you shatter that mirror reflection, that loving bond, then you grow up with no sense of self. You can't keep showing children themselves in warped and cracked mirrors and expect them to grow up normally. When they do get older, the warped mirrors are reinforced by society telling them that they are worthless, that they can't get a job or they belong in jail."

It wasn't until May 26, 1997, that the 680-page *Bringing Them Home: Report of the National Inquiry into the Separation of Aboriginal and Torres Strait Islander Children from Their Families* was tabled in the Australian Parliament by the Human Rights and Equal Opportunities Commission, finally acknowledging the country's dark colonial history and state-sanctioned genocide against the Indigenous peoples. Fifty-four recommendations were made, including apologizing for the sexual abuse many of the institutionalized children suffered. The apology was delivered by Prime Minister Kevin Rudd in 2008, more than a decade after the report was published.[11] The majority of recommendations have still not been fulfilled.

Today's Aboriginal youth are often born into a world characterized by normative instability, to parents who may have substance abuse issues, who live in extreme poverty or, because of their own disrupted upbringings, lack the tools necessary to raise children. They are born into social exclusion, so they are not only at risk of suicide, they also face higher rates of sexual abuse and of self-destructive behaviours such as petrol sniffing and other forms of substance abuse. According to an article in the *Guardian*, as of June 30, 2016, "Over half of the 16,767 Aboriginal and Torres Strait Islander children in care were living either with Indigenous kin or an Indigenous foster carer, while about a third remained with non-Indigenous carers to whom they were not related. The remainder were with non-Indigenous kin." And, the article continues, funding for mental health care, another recommendation, has not been relegated to Indigenous organizations or aimed at addressing the immediate and intergenerational trauma, "and [is] occasionally delivered by the same churches that were responsible for managing the missions."[12]

According to the 2017 annual *Closing the Gap* report, the country hit only one of the seven measures aimed at reducing the disadvantages and disparities in health, education, and employment among the Indigenous peoples.[13] In February 2018, a non-government group charged with reviewing *Closing the Gap* concluded that the government had "effectively abandoned" the policy.[14]

Helen calls the treatment of Aboriginal and Torres Strait Islanders a genocide, wherein the very essence of their existence was shattered: "Genocide takes place on many levels: physical, psychological, social, spiritual, and cultural. The sheer loss of physical life; the denial of identity and place in humanity; the fragmentation of families and the stealing of children; the denigration and destruction of entities most sacred; and the belittlement and vilification of culture occurred over generations. To stand on the edge of genocide is to stare into the abyss, to be lost forever." Genocide travels across time and in both directions, she says, separating us from the past and destroying our future hopes.

In the absence of any wide-scale mental health and wellness system, the onus is on the survivor, or the child or grandchild of the survivor, to find their way back. Many people have been unable to do that, Helen notes, because of the trauma they live with.

Profound trauma serves to isolate everyone

from each other and everything they know, leaving them in a state of disrepair, feeling lost and unknowing. The isolation, the loneliness of having no belonging, is almost like a force field that surrounds you; you can't reach out, and no one can reach in. You can't talk to anyone or bring anyone into your world of grief, and the only time you feel safe is when you are alone, when you are completely isolated and cut off from everyone else. These feelings shatter any chance of creating healthy human attachments. This is what it means to live life through the trauma lens.

"Think about all the people who love you in your life. They are like tethers to you. Cut the ties, and you have nothing to ground you. Not only do people not feel belonging, no one is holding on to the tethers to stop them from flying into the wind," Helen says. "Trauma shatters your future relationships or your ability to commit. You are so isolated, so why not kill yourself? It becomes a rational thought in this mind. You have no belonging, so you might as well go."

Helen speaks of living in the "third space." This space is best represented by one of her paintings, which she produced on her iPad while she was interviewing the victims of sexual abuse. One side of the painting is brightly coloured, and there is fluent movement, a synergy of flow and lines. This represents Aboriginal culture, she explains. On the other side, non-Aboriginal culture is represented by sharp, hard lines with little colour. The two sides of the painting almost come together in the middle, but they just can't. And that is the third space. The third space is the blank space.

"The kids are floating in the third space of trauma and loss and grief and despair, and it is not where they want to be," she says. "Until we clear out the third space, we can't move closer to healing."

TWENTY YEARS AGO, Mike Metatawabin first went to Wunnumin Lake First Nation to act as a Cree and Oji-Cree translator for the Elders coming inland from the James Bay coast to attend one of the summer NAN leadership meetings.

It was during this trip that Mike first met a Ralph Rowe survivor. The encounter altered the course of his life. He remembers sitting in the community hall and being overwhelmed by the odd, unsettling feeling that he needed to leave. He got up and walked away from the proceedings.

The cold rain soaked through his shoes as he

made his way to the modest cabin he was staying in. He hoped the wood stove would be on. But when he walked in, the cabin was dark and chilly, and he could feel someone's eyes on him. A young man was sitting in the corner. A small leather hand drum was on the table in front of him. The noose was near.

Mike took a seat and began to beat the drum. He told the young man of the pain he was holding after the sudden death of his infant just months earlier. The young man listened. Mike finished his story and continued to drum.

Then the young man spoke. He said that tonight was the night. He could not take it any longer. The hurt inside was unbearable, and no one seemed to care. He didn't feel as though he could talk to anyone in his community about what Ralph Rowe had done to him, because it was the community of the faithful who kept inviting the monster back, time and time again. Every time the Anglican priest flew into Wunnumin, he was met with praise and adulation. But the young man, who was then only a boy, knew what was in store for him. He was terrified and he couldn't tell anyone why. No one would believe that a revered man of the cloth would do such nasty things to a member of his flock.

The story poured out of the man, and Mike continued to drum. They sat together for hours, until they were both emotionally spent and Mike saw the danger pass from the man's eyes.

"I've never forgotten that moment. A time when someone was reaching out and I was the one who answered the call. It makes you wonder at the power of the will to live. At a time when all seems lost, an angel comes calling, sending a message to listen," Mike wrote in the Mushkegowuk Council of Cree Nations report *The People's Inquiry into Our Suicide Pandemic*.[15] Mike was the lead commissioner in the council's investigation of the suicide epidemic that was affecting the James Bay First Nations communities from Moose Cree to Attawapiskat to Fort Albany.

Following his encounter with the young man in Wunnumin in 1998, Mike would go on to extend his hand all across NAN territory, trying to find survivors who, for decades, had told no one about what had happened to them. He never dreamed that this encounter would lead to the discovery of hundreds of men, all survivors, living in the shadows with their pain, fighting their memories with alcohol, addiction, and violence, experiencing suicidal ideation, and in some cases dying by suicide. And Mike never dreamed that Rowe's legacy would continue to have an impact on the wives and the children of all of his victims.

To this day, the devastation of those assaults committed by a sick man echo like thunder in the twenty communities that were under the care of the flying Anglican priest. And his actions are linked to the deaths of the seven girls from Wapekeka and Poplar Hill First Nations four decades later.

ON THE WEB PAGE FOR Wapekeka First Nation, in small type down the left of the screen, there is a historical reference to the significance of the signing of Treaty No. 9 that echoes bittersweetly. It reads, "The sun coming up in the horizon at dawn, the river flowing ever so gently, the trees standing tall and grass from Mother Earth. One can hear the words of the Treaty Commissioner promising that the Queen will forever take care of her children. As long as the sun shines, as long as the river flows and as long as the grass grows."

Wapekeka First Nation is located about 450 kilometres northeast of Sioux Lookout, Northern Ontario. In 1929 the area was added as an adhesion to Treaty No. 9 as the province of Ontario expanded to the farthest northwest region, near the Manitoba border.[16] The only way to get to Wapekeka is by booking a charter flight (about $1,200 return) with Wasaya Airways, which is owned and operated by the First Nations it serves. Originally the Oji-Cree from Kitchenuhmaykoosib Inninuwug (KI), or Big Trout First Nation, used the lands here as a winter settlement, setting up traplines about twenty-six kilometres northwest of KI. Around that time, other communities left KI to settle in the surrounding area, at Kingfisher Lake, Wunnumin Lake, Bearskin Lake, Kasabonika, Muskrat Dam, and Sachigo.

Wapekeka was not officially registered as a band under the Indian Act until 1979. The English first called the community Angling Lake First Nation, but the Oji-Cree changed the name to Wapekeka. Nestled between Frog Lake and Angling Lake, it is made up of two reserve communities, Wapekeka 1 Indian Reserve and Wapekeka 2 Indian Reserve, and altogether occupies about fifty-two square kilometres. The land is rich with wildlife and endless freshwater lakes and has one of the last untouched areas of boreal forest left on Mother Earth.

In the dead of winter, the region is repressively cold, with stretches at minus thirty or forty degrees Celsius. When you breathe, the air exhaled from your lungs sticks in frozen droplets on any bits of exposed hair, even your eyelashes. The snow crunches, clean and white, under your feet. The only respite from the frigid conditions is to stay indoors, and there aren't too many places to go when you leave your house.

A dozen roads connect at the centre of the community, by a grey band office, a nursing station, an Ontario Provincial Police office, and an elementary school. The Reverend Eleazer Winter Memorial School burned down in May 2015 and reopened less than a year later, on February 3, 2016.[17] There is a small hotel, a grocery store, and the structural foundation for a new youth centre, covered by a large blue tarp to protect it from the elements. Construction on the youth centre has stalled because of the weather.

Wapekeka has three churches for a community of only 363 souls. Anglican is the dominant faith, and the Anglican Church's history in the community is complex. It has been both a saviour and, because of one man, a force of destruction. That man is a former priest named Ralph Rowe.

It is almost impossible to describe how damaging the actions of Ralph Knight Munck Rowe have been to the community of Wapekeka and the more than twenty other communities in Northwestern Ontario and in northern Manitoba. His cover was perfect. Rowe, the son of an Anglican clergyman, was first trained as an Ontario Provincial Police officer and sent to Manitoulin Island, an outpost in Georgian Bay that is home to a handful of First Nations communities. Around this time, he got involved with the Boy Scouts. He also took flying lessons.

Rowe abruptly left the police service, and in 1966 he moved to Kenora, Ontario, where he began to fly small charter flights to remote communities. From 1967 to 1970 he lived in Manitoba, where he devoted himself to theological study and became a lay reader for the Anglican Church, travelling in the summers to Weagamow and Neskantanga First Nations, living in each community for one month at a time. By 1971 he was living in Split Lake, Manitoba, and in 1975 he was ordained by the Anglican Church and charged with ministering to the remote First Nations communities of Northern Ontario.

Rowe endeared himself to people in the North who had adopted the Christian faith after their time in residential school. They saw Rowe as God's representative on Earth. He also took the time to learn Oji-Cree so he could talk to the Elders.

Rowe spent time in each community, taking special interest in young boys around the age of twelve. He took them on camping trips out in the bush and he became a Cub Scout leader, starting a program in Wunnumin Lake in 1977. Girls were never invited to his special outings with the boys. His method of operation was always the same, and he gained the trust and respect of all.

During Rowe's sentencing in Kenora in 2012, Justice D. Fraser described his actions as having a "bigger impact than even the residential school experience," because it was "fresher" and it affected a generation of men who were becoming leaders of their communities. "You were greatly respected, you drew young children to you like a pied piper and it is the confusion of that experience, somebody trusted and respected by parents, liked by children, and then suddenly turn[ed] into a parasite, a monster," Justice Fraser said. "If putting you through a mincing machine and feeding you to dogs would help, I would love to do that if that were in the Criminal Code but it is not and it would not help."[18]

From the 1970s until the mid-1980s, Rowe engaged in rampant sexual abuse of boys between the ages of eight and fourteen. It is estimated by NAN that Ralph Rowe's victims could number up to five hundred.[19] He is likely one of the country's most prolific pedophiles. But he has been charged with only about sixty sex crimes and has served no more than five years in prison, because of a plea bargain deal he made with the Crown.

Rowe now lives on Vancouver Island, in the small, sleepy community of Lake Cowichan. Journalist Stephanie Harrington visited Rowe at the local Anglican church, where he is a parishioner. Rowe says that he has been through "all kinds of programs" and "the fact is no one can be more sorry than I am." He also says he wants a "healing circle," something he has sought for the past thirty-one years. "And I've continued to be denied," he says. He maintains that there are many abuse claims, hundreds of them, that aren't true: "It's at a stage now where many things are included that really aren't true."[20]

Rowe's shadow hangs over the NAN communities. He has left a destructive legacy in communities that are already grappling with the after-effects of residential schools — broken marriages and families; physical and sexual abuse; violence and domestic assault; addiction issues; broken men with low self-confidence and confusing thoughts, coupled with the feeling they have nowhere to turn. The impact of these cases of child abuse, the trauma of the residential schools, and the poor living conditions on the reserves create a brutal cycle of shame. NAN Grand Chief Alvin Fiddler squarely blames Rowe for the suicides of dozens of adult men in their prime who were unable to cope with what he did to them, and for the cascading effect on the children or relatives of survivors.[21] Without proper on-site medical and mental health care in all the Northern communities, the situation is untenable.

Many who took their lives during the spike in suicides in Wapekeka First Nation in the 1990s were Ralph Rowe survivors. It was in response to that crisis that the community set up the annual Survivors of Suicide Conference, and it was within a year of its funding being cut in 2015 that the seven girls from Wapekeka and Poplar Hill First Nations died by suicide. And today the First Nations communities inside Treaty No. 9 — communities such as Pikangikum, Attawapiskat, Fort Albany, and Wapekeka — have one of the highest youth suicide rates in the Western world.

MPP Sol Mamakwa told me of a recent visit he made to the Thunder Bay hospital's psychiatric ward. Six girls had been medically evacuated from Wunnumin First Nation because of sexual assault. Sol knew one of the girl's families. "Every five minutes she would convulse. Her body was responding to the abuse," he said. "It was heartbreaking to watch."

There were three perpetrators in the community, all in their early twenties, and about twenty to twenty-five girls were affected. "The community has mixed feelings about the [most recent] suicide," said Sol. "He was one of the perpetrators of [the abuse of] the young girls."

Wunnumin Lake was one of the communities Rowe visited for years. In fact, it was a distant relative of Sol's, James Mamakwa, who in 1992 approached Ontario Provincial Police officer Don Hewitt (now retired) after hearing him speak at a community college in Thunder Bay, to tell him that he had been abused by Rowe. That led to the Wunnumin Lake investigation.[22]

After the immediate aid workers left Wapekeka in the wake of the girls' deaths — from the Junior Canadian Rangers, who were called in to walk the small, confined streets to check door-to-door on the youth, to trauma and mental health workers — the community hired four long-term mental health workers, another four youth workers, and four recreation support workers.

Anna Betty Achneepineskum says the multifaceted plan to address suicide and sexual abuse begins with Elder focus groups to get at the historical trauma, and then further focus groups with the women and men who lived in the community at the time. Band councillors and front-line workers will be trained in sexual boundaries, sexual trauma, and developing protocols for handling traumatic events. For instance, she says, when a young person loses a friend, what is the plan to deal with that loss? "The answer is not to send the child out of the community," she says; that is what children's aid societies have been doing, and it clearly does not work.[23]

Natan Obed, president of Inuit Tapiriit Kanatami, the national voice for sixty thousand Inuit who live in Canada, notes that leaders and Elders must be involved in conversations on controversial subjects like sexual abuse and gender-based violence. Children must be protected and deserve to have a happy, healthy childhood. "There is no way to talk about this issue without it being difficult," he says. "We need to do more to keep our children safe. We know the risk factor that child sexual abuse is for suicide."[24]

Sexual abuse is a main driver of high suicide rates in Indigenous communities across Canada, but it is not often talked about openly and confronted, notes the University of Saskatchewan's Jack Hicks. The suicide rate among young Indigenous women in the province between the ages of ten and nineteen is 29.7 times higher than that of non-Indigenous women in the same age range. The suicide rate among First Nations men in the same age group is comparatively 6.4 times higher than that of non–First Nations men.[25]

The *Saskatchewan First Nations Suicide Prevention Strategy*, the 2018 report for which Hicks served as technical consultant, asks poignant questions about the state of the girls' minds at the time of their deaths: "Given that teenaged First Nations girls in Saskatchewan have a sharply elevated rate of death by suicide, might they also have a sharply elevated rate of attempted suicide? If so, what might be the implications for these young women over their life courses? What might be the implications for the health system — what are these attempts costing the system? And fundamentally, what are the implications for society? At this point we have no idea."[26]

NO MATTER WHERE YOU ARE in Seabird, you can hear the long, mournful bellow of the train whistle. The Canadian Pacific Railway built a track directly through the reserve in 1881, two years after the founding of the community by the Indian Reserve Commission, which cleared space for migrating groups of First Nations who came together to settle on the land. Around the same time, the first community Roman Catholic church was established by the Missionary Oblates of Mary Immaculate.

Seabird is a modern, progressive community nestled in the lush green valleys of the Fraser River system in southern British Columbia, under the snow-capped near-pyramid of Mount Cheam. It has its own elementary and high schools, a vocational school, a daycare, and a thriving, well-staffed, and well-appointed medical centre. The centre permanently employs First Nations doctors and dentists and trained nurses.

Elder Maggie Pettis — who lost her brother, Cliff Pettis, to suicide five years ago, and then more recently her nephew, Brian Junior — has spent decades striving to improve health care and education at Seabird. She is now working on a suicide prevention study, funded by the federal government, on the need to return to land-based cultural teachings to bolster and strengthen Indigenous pride in each Seabird child. She believes her people are experiencing the fallout from the residential school system's forced disconnection of family and community, and now the routine apprehension of kids by child welfare officers. What follows are increases in addiction, mental health crises, high school dropouts, incarceration rates, and joblessness.

In the past several years, nearly half a dozen young men in the community of 1,150 have died by suicide on the railroad tracks. Each boy seemed to have a similar trigger — the breakup of a relationship or a fight or disagreement with a loved one. "Sometimes they are too far gone; their spirit is lost, and it is hard to pull them back," says Maggie.[27]

In 2016, Fraser Health, the University of the Fraser Valley, and Stó:lō Nation, a political tribal council consisting of eleven communities in the Fraser Valley area, applied for a Canadian Institute for Health Information research grant on youth suicide prevention for Seabird Island Nation. But Maggie says the program, while a necessary good start, falls well short of what is truly needed. "The process is too slow. We're losing people," she says.

Maggie knows everyone in Seabird, and she knows the struggles behind everyone's outward smiles. She hands out her cellphone number to community members in need of a sympathetic ear in times of personal crisis. When she sees Margo Jimmie and her seventeen-year-old daughter, Summer, at the health clinic, they both get an extra-warm greeting. On my visit to Stó:lō, Maggie introduces me to Margo so that I can hear her story.

For Margo it has been three years, and the pain inside has not subsided. She knows it never will. She is learning how to live with the hollowness of grief, and the road is not easy. Margo looks as if she has just walked out of a downtown Vancouver office tower. Her jet-black hair is fashionably short and swept to the side. When I meet her, she wears a thin black cotton cardigan over black pants and a blouse with a black, pink, and blue geometric print; large oval beaded earrings, bright blue and metallic, cover her earlobes and hang nearly halfway down her neck. Her long, hot-pink fingernails are filed into points, like talons. On her ring finger, instead of polish, a gold-and-diamond jewel is affixed to the nail.

Margo gets up every day and readies herself as if she were on her way to work. But she hasn't been to work for three years. Not since February 8, 2015. Not since her son, Bubbs, left her.

Margo raised Summer, Bubbs, and her other

son, Tristan, on her own after their father left. The children had no father figure in their lives until she met her current husband, nine years later. "It's hard for a boy to adjust when they have always only known Mom," she says. "So when a father figure comes in, it is hard for them to accept because they have no trust with males."

She remembers Bubbs as a loving child, charming, caring — but he struggled with mental health issues. She remembers that when he was five he had uncontrollable temper tantrums. But she thought it was normal, just a child of a single mom acting out.

She didn't have good relationships or frequent contact with doctors or nurses. Mental health services are hard to access. She remembers once taking Bubbs to the hospital due to a mental health episode. After waiting eight hours to see a psychologist, he left feeling even more isolated than before. He was exhausted and had just told her whatever she wanted to hear so he could leave. They were given a phone number and were told to call back if he got any worse.

"That doesn't work," scoffs Margo. "It works by sitting and talking and getting to the bottom of the issues. The person with mental health issues doesn't understand what is normal and what is not." She feels that mental health workers need to invest more time in the ones who are quiet and bottle everything up. Those teens aren't going to call for help.

Bubbs used to think someone was following him, so he couldn't stay in one place for too long. He could never explain who was coming after him. Whenever he had one of those episodes, no matter where he was, Margo would pick him up and bring him home.

"He wouldn't stay home for long. He'd take off. The more he'd take off, the more I'd find him. He'd get into relationships with girls. He already had a broken relationship with family members, and to go through a breakup with a girl was emotionally hard on him. I tried to explain to him that he would have many relationships in life and not all were going to stay. He had a whole life ahead of him," she says as the tears flow down her face.

But her words never got through to her son. And what happened next was stunning.

"Within the first year of his death, three of his friends passed away the same way," she says.

All suicides. All on the railroad tracks.

Bubbs left behind three children, two boys and a girl. Margo calls them her blessings.

Following her son's death, Margo shut off her phone. Then, for whatever reason, one day she turned it back on. As soon as she did, she got a call from the mother of Bubbs's friend Carlos.

"She said, 'Margo, I am at my doorway.' I asked if she was okay. She said, 'No, I am not okay. I am packing right now. I have the RCMP at my door and they just told me my son has gone to be with your son.' And I said, 'What do you say?' She said, 'My son is gone and I find myself standing here in the doorway. Can you come help me?' I said, 'I will call you right back.' I phoned my aunt and told her what had happened. I told her Carlos's mom was asking me to help her and I just didn't have the strength. I was already in a depression state at the time. I hadn't left the house for roughly six months. My aunt went over to help her. I am very fortunate my band was able to cover the family financially. And then we buried Carlos with my son."

Two more of Bubbs's friends died after that.

"Each time I would fall, and it has only been three years, and I tell you it has taken me this long to get here," she says. "I am still not back to work, but I make myself get up and leave the house as soon as everyone else leaves. But I have so many triggers at home, it is unbelievable. I knew suicide hit very [hard], and it has been my reality since Bubbs left. I carried a lot of self-blame for the first two years. What-ifs, how, what could have."

People who do not live in an Indigenous community cannot really grasp what it is like to grow up in an environment where suicide is the norm, where it is a part of everyday existence. For too many of these communities worldwide, life is lived immersed in the normalcy of death. But what's most alarming is the rate and frequency of suicide among youth. "Death is our life," says South Australian Elder Tauto Sansbury.[28]

Natan Obed knows what the impact of suicide feels like. As a hockey player and also as a coach in Nunatsiavut and Nunavut, Natan has lost count of how many hockey-playing peers or children — or parents of children he once coached — have died by suicide. Obed has been a driving force behind the creation of the National Inuit Suicide Prevention Strategy, which was released on July 27, 2016, in Knujjuaq, Nunavik. It is currently the only suicide prevention strategy in Canada that is co-ordinated on the national, regional, and community levels. Key to the program is identifying the common risk factors and creating "a shared, evidence-based, Inuit-specific approach to suicide prevention across

Inuit Nunangat."[29] He knows the risk factors are many, and they can begin in the womb with exposure to alcohol: the factors multiply if the child grows up in an overcrowded home or experiences malnutrition, food insecurity, neglect, or sexual abuse. If a parent or a close relative dies by suicide, the risk further increases.

According to Inuit Tapiriit Kanatami, people who go through stressful situations can react differently, depending on their coping skills and their family or community support. Protective factors are experiences, behaviours, or inherited characteristics that come from things like a stable home free of abuse, a strong connection to culture, and a solid education.[30] Without these stabilizing protective factors, a person is more vulnerable to the depression and anxiety that can lead to suicide.

The National Inuit Suicide Prevention Strategy identifies key priority areas: creating social equity, creating cultural continuity, nurturing healthy Inuit children from birth, ensuring access to a continuum of mental wellness services, healing unresolved trauma and grief, and mobilizing Inuit knowledge for resilience and suicide prevention.[31] What is clear is that at the heart of the suicides is a lack of the determinants of health and social equity — health care, housing, and a safe environment.

In the United States, it is estimated that Native American youth are "twice as likely to be exposed to domestic violence, sexual abuse, substance abuse, and poverty compared to other groups." Theresa M. Pouley, the chief judge of the Tulalip Tribal Court in Washington State, argues that these factors result in Indigenous youth developing post-traumatic stress disorder similar to that experienced by soldiers who served in Afghanistan.[32]

In Brazil, Indigenous people continue to be forcibly removed from their ancestral lands by domestic ranchers who often work for big multinational firms to produce crops such as sugar-cane, palm oil, and coffee. There are only 734,000 Indigenous people left in Brazil, accounting for 0.4 per cent of the country's population, down from nearly five million at the point of contact during the fifteenth century. There are only fifty-four Indigenous Nations left in Brazil.[33] To this day, Indigenous people face continued attacks, marginalization, and neglect in Brazilian society. Since 2007, 833 Indigenous people were murdered and, as noted in the previous chapter, more than 350 have died by suicide.[34]

Janete Morais, a Guarani law student at the Federal University of Rio Grande, comes from a reserve in northern Brazil that was set up before the 1988 constitutional change that strengthened Indigenous rights and environmental laws. She knows her people are lucky to have their own space and land; when she goes to school in the city, she passes by Guarani people living on streetsides or in the gutters. "They live on the roads," Morais says. "They don't have a place to live."

The Indigenous students and some professors at the university have been raising money to help the families survive. Morais says the continued trauma and societal marginalization wear down the will to live. "When something bad happens to them, their spirit becomes weak, and the first thing that comes to their mind is taking their own lives. They feel spiritually and psychologically weak," she says. There is a feeling of loss, a disconnection from the land. The constant fight to exist and to defend their territory, their abandonment by the government, the addiction issues all take their toll.

Morais, now thirty-five years old, thought about suicide many times when life became too difficult. But she says a strong spiritual connection to her grandfather, a shaman, kept her alive.[35]

Since the 1980s, researchers have also reported on the rise of suicide "clusters," defined as "serial suicides related in time, space, and etiology through a process of imitation."[36] When suicide becomes normalized in communities, it is an ever-present option, an alternative children live with while growing up seeing so many people around them dying. In North America, this phenomenon has occurred among the Hopi, Navajo, Pueblo, Flathead, and Wind River Nations, as well as in communities in Northern Ontario and among Inuit.[37] On April 10, 2016, seven children between the ages of nine and fourteen from the Northern Ontario community of Attawapiskat First Nation were admitted to the community's fifteen-bed hospital for possible drug overdoses in an attempted suicide. In all, there were eleven suspected suicide attempts within a twenty-four-hour period.[38]

There are also issues of underreporting or inaccuracies in reporting suicides among Indigenous populations, due to the lack of access to proper medical treatment, as well as a lack of epidemiological tracking by governments, with a few exceptions such as the Inuit in Canada.[39]

According to research in the *Canadian Journal of Psychiatry*, data taken from the 2008–10 First

Nations Regional Health Survey showed that exposure to a previous familial generation that went through residential school is associated with an "increased risk for lifetime suicide ideation." And having two generations of residential school history in your family increases the odds of "reporting a suicide attempt compared with having one generation." These findings show there are links between intergenerational exposure to residential school trauma, a higher risk of suicidal ideation, and a "cumulative risk in relation to suicide attempts across generations."[40]

Two of Canada's foremost researchers on youth suicide, the University of British Columbia's Michael Chandler and the University of Victoria's Christopher Lalonde, point out that among British Columbia's two hundred First Nations communities, it is estimated that Indigenous youth take their own lives at a rate between five and twenty times higher than that of non-Indigenous youth. Over the span of ten years, youth suicide rates varied in "wildly saw-toothed ways" from one community to another.[41]

Jack Hicks at the University of Saskatchewan believes Chandler and Lalonde's work should have taken a harder look at levels of community trauma and sexual abuse. He notes that Chandler and Lalonde used data collected between 1987 and 1992 from 196 of British Columbia's First Nations, and they found that 90 percent of youth suicides occurred in just 10 percent of the bands and that "some communities show rates some 800 times the national average while in others, suicide is essentially unknown."[42] However, suicide attempts, thoughts, or ideation was not measured.

"If it were found that no one living on that street died by suicide during a five-year period, would we therefore describe the street as one where 'suicide behaviour is essentially unknown'? Every human society we know of, present and past, experiences some degree of suicide behaviour. Why would Indigenous communities be otherwise?" Hicks asks. "Any very small population group may well go five or more years without a resident dying by suicide, but there will likely have been some amount of suicide ideation — and possibly suicide attempts."[43]

The socio-economic realities of many communities, along with adverse childhood events such as sexual abuse, cannot be removed from the equation.

MICHAEL CHANDLER AND Christopher Lalonde theorize that a large part of adolescent and teen development is a journey of self-discovery, a search for a sense of belonging.

All children struggle to find their identity, to discover who they are and where their place is in the world. But Indigenous youth are particularly weighed down by an inability to reconcile their personal and collective pasts, thus mitigating any sense of a viable future.[44] Without cultural or personal continuity with the past and the community, "life is easily cheapened and the possibility of suicide becomes a live option." If one's culture is "marginalized, or vandalized, or turned into a laughingstock," and if colonization has made one's community "criminalized, legislated out of existence or otherwise assimilated beyond easy recognition, then woe be upon those transiting toward maturity."[45]

Leslie Bonshor wanted to put Chandler and Lalonde's theory to the test. Bonshor is a member of Tzeachten First Nation, one of the communities that form Stó:lō Nation. Bonshor was the Aboriginal health director at Fraser Health when the Fraser Valley communities were experiencing a sudden spike in youth suicides. In 2012, seven

Stó:lō youths took their own lives within a six-month period, and there were far more attempts.[46] Around the same time, a suicide pact was discovered in East Vancouver — twenty-four children between the ages of twelve and fifteen were hospitalized for suicide risk. The youth suicides seemed to have become epidemic in southern BC.[47]

Bonshor noticed that the communities had all experienced a loss of connectiveness, a black hole in their history when everything was taken away — culture, language, children. She kept thinking that maybe Chandler and Lalonde were right; if she and her colleagues could get a community to function proudly, steeped in its culture, heritage, and language, they could reduce the suicide rates among the youth. Bonshor found a BC youth suicide strategy and went to work Indigenizing it specifically for the Fraser Valley area, including Seabird.

The scooping of children from their families and then placing them with white foster families has been a prevailing issue in Canada, just as it is in Australia, and there are also reports that this is happening with increasing frequency in Brazil. Today there are more Indigenous kids in the child welfare system than were enrolled in residential schools at their height. The term "Sixties Scoop" was coined by Patrick Johnston in his book, *Native Children and the Child Welfare System*, in which he documented a conversation he had with a retired social worker from BC who said that the children were routinely "scooped" from their parents. She and her colleagues honestly thought they were helping the kids. By the time Johnston interviewed the social worker, she tearfully admitted it had been a terrible mistake.[48]

By the early 1950s, the federal government had stopped making it mandatory for Indigenous children to attend residential school. But authorities still believed that the children needed to be educated and the role should fall to the provincially run public school system. But the children did not live near the schools. In 1951, the federal government amended the Indian Act to allow provinces the ability to provide services such as child welfare and protection to their Indigenous communities. And the provinces were allocated funding to do so. Lots of it.[49]

The 1960s saw an explosion of kids into the child welfare system. Child welfare workers who had no training in or knowledge of Indigenous culture began to take children from their families and place them in foster care. The workers compared how children were being raised in First Nations homes to their own Euro-Canadian ways and values. So if they entered homes where the food was all wild game, berries, and vegetables, where they saw the poverty, addictions, and other social ills of reserves, they assumed the kids were in danger and took them away — often without informing anyone in the community. In BC, for example, it wasn't until 1980 that social workers were required to notify the band council when an Indigenous child was taken into state custody.[50]

As a result, children not only suffered the trauma of being separated from their parents and communities, they also experienced a sudden rupture from their culture and damaging disruption of the development of their identities.[51]

The scooping of children exists to this day. Assembly of First Nations Chief Perry Bellegarde estimates forty thousand Indigenous children are currently in state care. Less than 8 percent of all kids in Canada under the age of four are Indigenous, but they represent 51.2 percent of preschoolers in foster care. The federal minister responsible for Indigenous services in Canada, Jane Philpott, calls the current system "perverse." Instead of perpetuating the apprehension of at-risk children, she says, the system should focus on preventing family problems. In January 2018, she introduced a six-point plan that focuses on keeping families together.[52]

Spensy Pimentel, a Brazilian journalist and anthropologist at the Federal University of Southern Bahia, says Indigenous children are being taken from their families and placed with white families with increasing frequency. "When we have an economic crisis and families don't have jobs, they use breadbaskets and food banks," Pimentel says. "But those programs are being cut and the authorities take the kids and give them to white people to adopt. This is a cultural problem."[53]

All colonized communities grapple with intergenerational trauma. From 1850 to roughly 1980, the Sami suffered from policies of assimilation that were developed to consolidate the emergence of nation-states, especially in Norway with the introduction of "Norwegianization." In the nineteenth century, such "harmonization policy" was not unique. In Finland and in the Baltic states, there was a policy called "Russification," and in Central Europe the Prussian statesman and first chancellor of Germany, Otto von Bismarck, introduced "Germanification." Later, during the Cold War era, the policy of assimilation was justified as a security measure.[54]

For more than a century, Norway concentrated efforts on assimilating the Sami. The cornerstone of the policy was to achieve ethnic cleansing through the eradication of language and culture, and re-education and indoctrination through the Norwegian school system and the adoption of Christianity. Harald Eidheim, a founder of Norwegian social anthropology and one of the foremost scholars on the Sami, particularly during the postwar years, argued that one of the most significant issues affecting the Sami in Norway was the public's perception of the people, who were regarded as "beggarly, old-fashioned, reactionary, and — in many circles — heathen." As a result of the shame they experienced at school, which was reinforced by society at large, the Sami hid their culture and traditions.[55] Still today, the negative stereotypes and insensitive representation persist. In 2015, Finnair and VisitFinland produced an advertisement depicting Sami in traditional clothing, dancing around a fire during a shamanistic ritual. The actors were not of Sami origin and the setting and props were inauthentic. Following objections on social media, the video was taken down from

the Internet.[56] As a result of these negative projec-
tions, the Sami people suffer from the same sense
of powerlessness, hopelessness, and negative self-
image as other marginalized Indigenous Nations.[57]

"Tell them we don't just wander around" is
a famous remark made by a Sami herder to the
British-Canadian ethnographer Robert Paine, who
researched the Sami for fourteen years during the
1950s and 1960s.[58]

Simon Issát Marainen, poet and famous singer
of traditional Sami songs called *joik*, was called
home to manage the family herd of nearly thirteen thousand reindeer when his brothers Gustu
and Heaika, twenty-nine and twenty-one years
old respectively, died by suicide in the same year.
Gustu, the family's main reindeer herder, took
his life in early January 2014; Heaika followed in
November.[59]

Simon remembers Gustu, the happy-go-lucky
one, telling him he would never do that, that it
would never happen. But ultimately he decided to
end his life, alone among the reindeer, high up in
the hills.

Now Simon finds himself on an ATV in the summer and a snowmobile in the winter, motoring
alongside the herd over the valleys and fjords. "I

had never been 100 percent with the reindeer, but I had to take over, and now I am with them every day," he says. "I had a dream to make a career of my music, to travel all over the world, and I have been all over. I have been to Europe, Botswana, China, with my band, but I don't have that opportunity anymore." Now he has a young family of three children.

The life of a reindeer herder is not easy. The animals do not know international borders, and Norway is trying to discourage the herders from moving along their traditional path north, from the Swedish territories up to the coast. The Norwegian government has historically imposed fines on herders who trespass on private property. Simon's family has received fines of $575,000 Norwegian kroner ($93,000 Canadian). The government is also selling the herding land to developers to build cottages for European vacationers.

"We need this land for our animals. Without the land we can't live," Simon says. "My mom and dad are really worried. My parents are older now. I have two sisters but they don't work with the reindeer. Our whole family is pressured from all sides. There is a big fight to live the Sami life. There isn't anyone who believes in the reindeer herders; no one trusts us. My oldest brother, he was always so positive, so glad and happy, and then one day he was just gone. He finished his life when he was among the reindeer herd.

"But you can't give up on your life, on your culture," he says. "You belong to something, and without this we are nothing."

FOUR

"I BREATHE FOR THEM"

ON JANUARY 22, 2018, a snowstorm raged outside, while inside the Wabano Centre for Aboriginal Health in Ottawa, a forum of First Nations, Inuit, and Métis youth had been brought together by We Matter, a national Indigenous-led non-profit organization started by a sister-and-brother team from Hay River, Northwest Territories. The Attawapiskat suicide crisis in James Bay had motivated Tunchai and Kelvin Redvers to establish the youth empowerment group. Using a social media model similar to the It Gets Better Project in the United States, which offers LGBTQ+ youth support, We Matter uses multimedia — videos, art, writing — to send positive messages to youth from Indigenous role models and allies.

The Wabano Centre provides holistic, culturally relevant health services to First Nations, Inuit, and Métis communities of Ottawa and is housed in a beautiful twenty-five-thousand-square-foot building designed by renowned Indigenous architect Douglas Cardinal. A majestic stone staircase leads up to a smooth curvilinear structure, Cardinal's signature. The main floor, called the Water Floor, contains prenatal and primary care clinics and a Cedar Lodge used for sweats. Walk up the stairs to the second floor, the Fire Floor, and you'll see a giant domed ceiling featuring a beautiful medicine wheel illuminated by a skylight. Look down and you'll see that the red- and earth-toned floor tiles are shaped in the pattern of a Star Blanket. The Star Blanket is traditionally given to honour people at pivotal stages of life, such as birth or marriage. If you stand at the centre of the star and speak out, your voice echoes throughout the room.

The Fire Floor features Wabano's Grand Gathering Space, and this is where nearly ninety youth had gathered together with politicians — including the national chief of the Assembly of First Nations, Perry Bellegarde, and Canada's Indigenous Services minister, Jane Philpott — and representatives of Facebook to talk about how suicide had affected the youth and their communities. Facebook is a prominent tool of communication in isolated Indigenous communities, and the social media powerhouse was in attendance because of its unique capability of detecting suicidal behaviour online. A microphone was passed around the circle.

Jenna, from a Mi'kmaq community in Halifax, told the group she had recently lost her cousin, who had struggled with anxiety and depression: "He was a mixed martial arts fighter, twenty years old, a firefighter. He reached out. If we had culturally appropriate mental health care, I think he'd still be here today. He took his life after he was given a two-month wait time [for treatment]. We can't stop fighting."

Lori, also a Mi'kmaq from Nova Scotia, said, "A lot of us here have undergone trauma — sexual violence, violence, abuse — from family members, people who are supposed to be our friends."

Matthew, a Haida Gwaii youth from British Columbia, called suicide the darkness "bringing us down. I have thought about it more than once. We all have one thing in common: we are all suffering. My thirteen-year-old sister ran away. We have fear and shame that we all hide. We need to hope again. Think of our loved ones, our future, our families."

Cody, an Ojibwe youth who grew up in Ottawa, said, "I see the poverty that is here. I see our people struggling on the street. I actively used drugs and alcohol for years. I am twenty-five years old and I just met my relatives last year. It took me twenty-four years to meet my family. Growing up, I felt inferior, dirty, like I didn't belong here. But being brought into a healing circle by Elders and good medicine got me here."

Dalton, from Midland, Ontario, talked about the loss of his best friend: "Two years ago, I attempted. My parents knew. I went for a walk one day in the bush and my best friend followed me. I tried to overdose. But because of her, I didn't. She is the reason why I am here today. But she did it. Last year, my best friend took her own life. I struggle every day."

Dakota, a young First Nations paramedic from Northern Saskatchewan, said young people often call 911 when they are feeling suicidal. "They call us for help. Some of them are brought in [to the hospital] for help and are let out two hours later. Why [do] the hospitals accept these kids and let them out? I want to create places for them close to home." Dakota pauses before he continues: "I work CPR on young people. I breathe for them."

EVERY INDIGENOUS NATION HAS its own holistic healing practices, traditions, and medicine people that for centuries it has relied on to take care of body, mind, and spirit — all of which, in the Indigenous worldview, are connected. The medicine man or healer acts as a spiritual leader and counsellor, responsible for individuals' physical, spiritual, and mental health as well as the community's social well-being. If someone is sick, the whole person is treated. By contrast, Western medicine isolates mental, spiritual, and physical treatment. Even the body is divided, with a specialist for each part.[1]

Those connections to their holistic home cultures and knowledge were severed when Indigenous people were forcibly removed from their land and resettled in remote areas, when they were taken away from their families and sent to residential schools or foster care, when they were quarantined and confined to Indian hospitals, when they experienced racist and discriminatory behaviour from doctors and nurses. And as a result, Indigenous people in Canada and beyond have developed a genuine mistrust of the Western health system.

For a decade between 1942 and 1952, Dr. Percy Moore, branch superintendent of medical services for the Department of Indian Affairs, and Dr. Frederick Tisdall, president of the Canadian Paediatric Society and one of three pediatricians at the Hospital for Sick Children who developed the baby cereal Pablum, performed nutritional experiments on children in six residential schools. Ian Mosby, a food historian, exposed details of these experiments, including malnourishment of the children to see if supplements such as riboflavin and thiamine would provide adequate nutrition. They did not. Parents were not informed of the experiments conducted on their children, and the researchers continued their work even as children died. This happened during the Nuremberg trials, at which twenty Nazi doctors were convicted for violating the Hippocratic Oath, resulting in the release of the Nuremberg Code of Medical Ethics in 1946.[2]

"This research gives some insight into the mindset of these colonial administrators from the federal government and the way they thought of Aboriginal people," Mosby said in an interview on CBC Radio in 2013. "The fact that they saw them as someone who could be used as experimental materials in their own research shows an ideology at work here."[3]

In Australia, Aboriginal people and Torres Strait Islanders are reluctant to access health care because of the lack of culturally appropriate care and the fear that entering the medical system will result in their removal from the community.[4] The distrust of government institutions is well documented in the damning report released by the Royal Commission into Institutional Responses to Child Sexual Abuse. Aboriginal and Torres Strait Islander survivors told the commissioners about the abuse they suffered in residential institutions and missions, which they described as violent environments in which they were routinely humiliated, their culture and identity undermined, and where physical, emotional, and sexual violence was normalized. The abuse also extended to youth detention centres and out-of-home placements.[5]

At the turn of the twentieth century, "lock hospitals" were established on Bernier and Dorre Islands in Australia, under the guise of treating Aboriginal women for venereal disease — an idea that originated in England, where women who were believed to be prostitutes were locked away in garrison hospitals under the Contagious Diseases Act. Melbourne and Brisbane had lock hospitals for women thought to be prostitutes. On Bernier and Dorre Islands, it was Aboriginals and Torres Strait Islanders who were held captive, often having been forcibly removed from their homes. There they were subjected to invasive treatments and suffered high death rates. According to Dr. Robin Barrington, a Yamaji Aborigine researcher, the hospitals were "places of imprisonment, exile, isolation, segregation, anthropological investigations and medical experiments made possible by laws of exception."[6]

The Australian government acknowledges that accessing social services is sometimes a traumatic experience for Indigenous people because of past associations with substandard health care provision, the removal of children, and generally discriminatory treatment, all of which discourage Aboriginal people and Torres Strait Islanders from seeking treatment until a crisis occurs.[7]

Hospital care for mental health issues can be a "particularly inappropriate" response for Aboriginal peoples and Torres Strait Islanders, especially for those living in rural areas. A study of Aboriginal peoples in central Australia reported that 90 percent wanted alternatives to hospital care, compared with 47 percent of non-Aboriginal people. Leaving their home communities to receive care at city hospitals only added to the trauma.[8]

About two-thirds of the American Indian and Alaskan Native population live in urban centres, yet one-third do not have a doctor or access to a clinic. One-third of Native Americans don't have health insurance, compared to 11 percent of white Americans.[9] The federal government, through the Indian Health Service (IHS), is the main provider of health services for Native Americans who belong to one of the 573 recognized tribes. The IHS provides "comprehensive" health coverage for 2.2 million of 3.7 million Indigenous people. The life expectancy of Native Americans is 5.5 years less than that of the non-Native population, and the American Indian and Alaskan Native people lead less healthy lives because of "inadequate education, disproportionate poverty, discrimination in the delivery of health services, and cultural differences. These are broad quality of life issues rooted in economic adversity and poor social conditions."[10]

The conditions that people are born into, where they live, how they grow and learn and age — all of these play a factor in their overall health.[11] Without income, employment, food, shelter, and social equity, Indigenous children live without a sense of security, without a sense of their human dignity.

DR. MIKE KIRLEW MEETS ME at the Sioux Lookout Airport because it is minus forty degrees and my rental car won't start. During the winter months in Sioux Lookout, cars need to be plugged into power outlets overnight or their batteries will freeze. Mike laughs as he tries to jam the key into the ignition of the Toyota-turned-ice-block, but the key won't move. The steering wheel won't budge. Everything is frozen.

The sun blazes in the cloudless blue sky, but it gives us no warmth as we scurry over to his car and hop inside. Mike takes off his thick, beautifully beaded moose-hide mitts and pushes back his beaver fur hat before he starts the car and turns up the seat warmers. He pops in some Bob Marley. The smooth sounds of reggae evoke images of a climate about eighty degrees warmer, a perfect antidote to the harsh realities of the Canadian winter.

Mike is a physician who has devoted his entire life to living and working in Sioux Lookout. He arrived here by fluke — he had hoped to go to Moose Factory, along the James Bay coast, but he was told the medical residency program was full and instead he had to go to the Sioux. For nearly eleven years, Mike has been grappling with the suicide crisis in Northern Ontario, and he sees no end in sight. He is the one who, on a moment's notice, drops everything to fly up on a medical transport in the middle of a minus-forty-degree winter night to respond to a health crisis in Canada's remote North. He cared for Jolynn Winter and Chantell Fox in Wapekeka when they were toddlers. He sees first-hand how a lack of the determinants of health — education, basic services, a safe environment, and employment — debilitates these communities.

"Let me take you on the five-dollar tour of town," he says, then laughs before correcting himself: "Okay, maybe it's the $4.99 tour."

Sioux Lookout, Ontario, is a modest town of nearly five thousand people located halfway between Thunder Bay and Winnipeg, high up on the Canadian Shield, nestled among lakes and river systems that extend from Hudson Bay in the north to the Gulf of Mexico in the south, the Columbia River in the west, and the St. Lawrence in the east. Carbon dating of charcoal in the area has uncovered evidence that Sioux Lookout has been home to various First Nations for the past eight thousand years.[12] Sioux Lookout gets its name from the top of a hillside near Pelican Lake. As the story goes, the Ojibwe who lived around Gichigami, or Lake Superior, were always under attack from the Sioux, who lived on the western plains. One day, the Ojibwe devised a plan. When their lookout spotted the Sioux on Frog Rapids from a high peak of land, he sent out a warning to those who had set up camp below. When the Sioux landed on the beach, the Ojibwe ambushed them, and a great battle ensued. All but one little Sioux boy were drowned or killed.[13]

Sioux Lookout today is a picturesque town full of American fishermen and adventurers in the summer, and forestry and health care workers all year round. Throughout the day, float planes land on Pelican Lake and pickup trucks form a constant ring past the drive-through window at the Tim Hortons. But the best coffee and home-baked goods can be found at Roy Lane Coffee, on Sioux Lookout's main drag, sleepy Front Street, also known as First Avenue North, depending on which direction you're travelling. The town's quiet is broken only by the frequent sound of trains rumbling along the Canadian National Railway's transcontinental main line. Lac Seul First Nation, made up of three communities — Frenchman's Head, Kejick Bay, and Whitefish Bay — is located about forty kilometres outside of town.

We turn up Seventh Avenue and park the car

beside an institutional-looking cream-coloured low-rise building, boarded up and covered in No Trespassing signs. We step out onto the frozen snow and walk up to the entranceway, which still has a sign posting clinic hours.

This is the old Zone Hospital, Mike tells me. He pauses for a minute and then says, "This is the Indian hospital."

In the 1920s, the government began to establish segregated Indian hospitals. Many community and city hospitals refused to treat Indigenous patients or relegated them to separate wards, basements, and poorly ventilated areas. The patients were often treated as "indigents," unwanted burdens on the community, never a part of the greater society.[14]

In the nineteenth and early twentieth centuries, missionaries from various religious orders established Indian tuberculosis sanitoriums, which were taken over by the government and later converted to general hospitals for Indigenous people.[15] For nearly a century, the prevailing belief was that TB became more virulent when an Indigenous person was infected with the disease. According to the Canadian Public Health Association, in the 1930s and 1940s TB death rates were seven hundred per one hundred thousand, among the highest ever reported. The death rate from TB among children living in residential schools was even worse, with eight thousand deaths per one hundred thousand kids.[16] Residential school children lived in a constant state of neglect, inadequately clothed and fed. When they complained of feeling ill, they were often ignored, or they were sent to the school nursing station, which routinely failed to provide proper medication or adequate care.

In 1907, Dr. Peter Bryce, the chief medical officer of Canada, visited thirty-five residential schools and found them overcrowded, unsanitary, and poorly ventilated. In the resulting *Report on the Indian Schools of Manitoba and the North-West Territories*, he noted, "Of a total of 1,537 pupils reported upon nearly 25 percent are dead, of one school with an absolutely accurate statement, 69 percent of ex-pupils are dead, and that everywhere the almost invariable cause of death given is tuberculosis." He laid blame for the horrendous death rates on the churches and government officials running the schools.[17]

Duncan Campbell Scott, the superintendent of Indian Affairs, confirmed that he knew the children were dying in record numbers from the disease. Still, he refused Bryce's repeated requests for aid:

"It is readily acknowledged that Indian children lose their natural resistance to illness by habituation so closely in residential schools and that they die at a much higher rate than in their villages. But this does not justify a change in the policy of this Department which is geared towards a final solution of our Indian Problem." Scott then went on a campaign to undermine Bryce, pulling his funding and attempting to ruin his reputation and career. In 1921, Bryce was forced out of the government.[18]

In Sioux Lookout, the Indian hospital opened in 1949 and was in use until 1998. "It was a modern-day apartheid here," Mike says. *Apartheid* is an Afrikaans word meaning "apartness."[19] In 1913, the South African government passed the Native Land Act, which segregated Black South Africans by relegating them to reserves. It also became illegal for them to farm.[20] This racist policy gave rise to the opposition South African National Native Congress, which was renamed the African National Congress in 1923. In 1948, the South African National Party took power and passed a series of apartheid laws — prominent among them the Population Registration Act, which kept a government record of the population classified by racial group: Bantu (Black), coloured (mixed race), Asian

(Indian or Pakistani), or white. Laws and privilege flowed from there. Black people lived in segregated communities, were forbidden from entering some public institutions, had lower educational standards, and had to have a pass to travel into white communities.[21] According to some scholars, South African legislators had actually gone to Canada to study the Indian Act before implementing many aspects of apartheid.[22]

The history of the Indian hospitals proves that the health and well-being of Indigenous people in Canada was never — and I will argue is still not — equal to that of non-Indigenous Canadians. Indian hospitals arose, in part, because local hospitals did not want to admit, or pay for the care of, Indigenous tuberculosis patients. In an effort to contain the spread of the disease, Canada's Department of Indian Affairs reluctantly began to open separate hospitals to treat the Indigenous people. By the 1960s, there were twenty-two fully functioning Indian hospitals across the country.[23]

In the early twentieth century, racially segregated hospitals, and wards or wings within hospitals, proliferated in Western Canada, and not just for Indigenous patients. Chinese and Japanese patients had their own ward, "Ward H," in the Vancouver General Hospital. In the 1940s, Chinese TB patients were sent to Vancouver's St. Joseph's Oriental Hospital, where they were made to clean the toilets, they received little nursing care, and those on their deathbeds were routinely converted to Christianity.[24]

A number of horrors and abuses took place in the Indian hospitals. Not only were Indigenous people quarantined from the general white population, patients were admitted and confined in order for the hospitals to get increased funding — the longer the patients stayed, the more money the hospital received from the federal government.[25] Often staff did not have proper qualifications, and facilities were set up in old army barracks or other buildings that were not designed to function as medical institutions. In the 1930s, the federal government discovered that medical care at the Fort Qu'Appelle Indian Hospital in Saskatchewan and the Dynevor Indian Hospital in Manitoba could be delivered at half the cost of a regular community hospital, which led to the establishment of even more Indian hospitals.[26]

The conditions in these institutions were universally horrific. The hospitals were overcrowded with patients suffering from TB and a host of other contagious illnesses and infections. One doctor called a ward full of women and children a "pest house" and felt that the patients were better off at home.[27] Hospitals struggled to find nurses, who were usually poorly paid and overburdened with patients; one hospital had one nurse for seventy-five beds.[28]

In addition, harmful medical experimentation and questionable therapies were practised on patients. From 1949 to 1953, doctors at the Charles Camsell Indian Hospital outside of Edmonton performed 374 experimental surgeries, all under local—not general—anesthetic, to treat TB.

One sixteen-year-old Blackfoot patient watched doctors remove three of his ribs. "They used a saw. I was awake and I could hear the saw," he later recounted. "They got part way and then they told me, 'Now we are breaking the ribs off.'" He also remembered they scraped three other ribs and extracted a part of his lung, then used wax in the cavity to hold everything together.[29]

Surgery was painful and left many patients deformed. In Manitoba, the Sanitorium Board reported, "One-third of the patients died, one-third half recovered, and one-third were cured."[30]

In the 1940s, in Prince Rupert, British Columbia,

a group of petitioners calling themselves the Community Council Association requested the establishment of an Indian hospital to protect the local population from Natives with TB or venereal disease. At the subsequently established Miller Bay Hospital, female TB patients were forbidden from going outside, and windows were kept shut because the mechanisms used to open them were broken. The boys' ward had twenty-six beds, one toilet, and no windows.[31]

Medical abuses and experiments were also practised on children. In Fort Qu'Appelle Indian Hospital, drug tests for the BCG tuberculosis vaccine were performed on infants without parental consent. And young children who misbehaved or who would not lie still in their beds were physically restrained; in some instances their legs were put in casts so they couldn't move.[32]

In 1953, the Indian Act was amended so that if an Indigenous person refused to see a doctor or go to a hospital, or attempted to leave the hospital before being discharged or without the proper authorization, they would be charged with committing a crime.[33] According to author Bob Joseph of the Gwawaenuk Nation, a provision still remains in the act that says the government may make regulations to "provide compulsory hospitalization and treatment for infectious diseases among Indians."[34]

TB spread to the Inuit in the 1950s, with the arrival of the Hudson's Bay Company and the accompanying settlers. In that decade alone, one-third of the population was infected with it. From 1950 to 1969, health care workers made their way to Inuit territory to perform medical examinations. Inuit who were infected were taken to hospitals in the south. By 1956, one-seventh of the Inuit population was in southern Canada, receiving care. According to the Canadian Public Health Association, "Some were never seen again."[35]

If a patient died in hospital, their family was responsible for paying the cost of transporting the body home for burial. Many could not afford the expenditure, and to this day, the bodies of their loved ones rest in unmarked graveyards far from home.

WHILE MOST OF THE Indian hospitals were shuttered in the 1960s, Indigenous people continued to receive inadequate treatment. In 1988, Josias Fiddler, who at the time was chief of Sandy Lake First Nation in Northern Ontario, staged a hunger strike with four others from his community — Peter Goodman, Allan Meekis, Peter Fiddler, and Luke Mamakeesic — to protest the substandard treatment of the twenty-eight surrounding First Nations communities at the Sioux Lookout Zone Hospital as a result of deteriorating relations with the Canadian government's Health and Welfare branch. Of the eighteen thousand people living in the area, only four thousand were not Indigenous,[36] yet members of the community complained of inadequate translation services, poor treatment by staff, and frequent delays of emergency medical transports. "There were a lot of frustrations," Fiddler told the *Wawatay News*.[37]

The two-day hunger strike prompted a report that examined conditions within the communities and patient treatment provided by the hospital. Completed in 1989 by Wally McKay, a former grand chief of Nishnawbe Aski Nation; Dr. Harry Bain, the pediatrician-in-chief at the Hospital for Sick Children in Toronto; and Anglican archbishop Edward Scott, the report noted rising "racial tensions" in the area as a result of the increased number of First Nations people who had come to Sioux Lookout for school, work, and health care.[38] It also pointed to family breakdowns within the communities due to the residential school experience, a loss of traditional spirituality, a serious rise in mental health issues, and "alarming" rates of youth suicide.[39]

The probe recommended the creation of a single regional hospital. It also recommended that by 1995, the surrounding First Nations communities be given access to clean water and proper sewage treatment and power systems. (That is still far from a work in progress.)

By 1997, all four parties — Nishnawbe Aski Nation, the Municipality of Sioux Lookout, the Province of Ontario, and the federal government — had come to an agreement on the new hospital. In 2010, the Sioux Lookout Meno Ya Win Health Centre opened its doors. The hospital board was made up of five First Nations people, five people from the town, two doctors, and a traditional healer.[40] The sixty-bed hospital included a circular healing room constructed from cedar. The ceiling was painted in equal parts red, white, yellow, and black, representing the Anishinaabe four directions, and is specially ventilated so sage and sweetgrass can be burned for smudging, a traditional ceremony that cleanses or purifies one's body, mind, and spirit and the ceremonial space.

A new hundred-bed hostel for patients flying in from the North, and for those who need detoxification services, is attached to the hospital. The beautiful brand-new facility is located just down the street from the old Indian Hospital, which Mike Kirlew passes daily on his way to work. "It is a constant reminder of colonization's grip," he says.

The health system in Northern Ontario is still in crisis. And it isn't just Northern Ontario; the United Nations special rapporteur on the rights of Indigenous peoples says the crisis exists throughout Canada, and significant improvements in funding and policy changes are desperately needed.[41] The need for relief and change is overwhelming.

Toronto addiction medicine specialist and family physician Dr. Alexander Caudarella and his partner, pediatrician Dr. Andrea Evans, spend nearly four months of every year in Iqaluit. When they were in medical school at McGill University, the other doctors talked about taking their medical skills to remote areas around the world. Alexander and Andrea, by contrast, talked about going to Nunavut, and when the opportunity presented itself, they jumped at it and never looked back. A large part of what they deal with is suicide and attempted suicide. They wish they had more time to work on prevention; instead, they mostly confront the aftermath. "It has been eye-opening," Alexander says. "We thought we had an understanding about the world we live in."[42] But they soon realized they did not.

Alexander and Andrea know it is critical they reach out to children between the ages of nine and fifteen. "They have seen so much multi-generational trauma," Alexander says. Suicide has become part of their lives; it is normalized, part of the everyday lexicon. "The language of suffering becomes the language of suicidality. We hear often, 'My uncle killed himself, and so did my grandfather,' and some youth say that this is just what you do."

But community members are starting to open up and talk about suicide, which Alexander says is a positive step forward. Solutions will have to be Inuit-generated and -led. "The best solutions and ideas are coming from these same communities, these same elders and children. What is wonderful is that people are starting to listen."

Article 24(2) of the UN Declaration on the Rights of Indigenous Peoples states that Indigenous people have the right to access the same standard of health care as non-Indigenous people,[43] but in many colonized nations that protocol has not been fulfilled. In Australia, one-quarter of Indigenous youth have reported a long-term ailment or condition such as asthma, hearing loss, or skin problems. And 20 percent of Aboriginal young people living in urban areas report hearing loss due to an inflammatory disease called otitis media, severe ear infections linked to poverty. Impaired hearing affects language comprehension and school performance and can lead to behavioural issues. A housing shortage also makes it challenging to raise stable families and contributes to the intervention of child welfare services. A government survey revealed that 95 percent of Indigenous people in Australia live in private dwellings, and three-quarters of them are rentals. "I live on Social Security and I have two children who are in high school," one Aboriginal parent said. "It is hard enough for our children to stay at school but when they have to move from school to school because we need to move and have a roof over our heads, it is very unsettling for them."[44]

In Brazil, Indigenous children continue to live in severe poverty, and they often die from preventable causes. According to a 2015 UNICEF report, Indigenous children are twice as likely as others to die before they reach the age of one. And the majority of the more than three million children and adolescents who are not in school are from Indigenous or Afro-Brazilian communities.[45]

In Brazil's Mato Grosso do Sul region, UNICEF reported in 2005 that twenty-five Indigenous children belonging to the Guarani-Kaiowá tribe died of malnutrition, and in a situation similar to Northern Ontario's, young children are dying from preventable diseases and many suffer from anemia. Nils Kastberg, UNICEF's regional director for Latin America and the Caribbean, said the malnutrition is particularly objectionable, given that Latin America is a breadbasket of the world: "Latin America produces more food per person than most other parts of the world, which makes it even more unacceptable for children to be dying of hunger and malnutrition."[46]

In Canada, half of all First Nations children live in poverty, the life expectancy of First Nations people is five to seven years less than that of other Canadians, and the practice of placing Indigenous children in foster care remains a significant issue. Secondary school graduation rates for First Nations youth living on reserve are at 35 percent, compared to 85 percent for non-Indigenous kids. The TB rate is still 31 percent higher in Indigenous communities, and suicide rates are five to seven times the national average.[47]

Indigenous people are overrepresented in the prison system. One-quarter of all adults and youth incarcerated in Canada are Indigenous.[48] Incarceration rates are similarly high in Australia, where Aboriginal people and Torres Strait Islanders make up 27 percent of the inmate population but only 3 percent of the country's total population.[49]

In addition, Indigenous inmates are often subject to inhumane treatment. On December 29, 2015, twenty-six-year-old David Dungay Jr., an Aboriginal man who was diabetic and had mental health issues, died after being tackled by prison guards in a Sydney jail and pinned to his bed. The incident was caught on video. On it he is heard gasping, "I can't breathe, please!" He made the plea twelve times before perishing.[50]

In 2016, Ontario Human Rights Commissioner Renu Mandhane was tipped off by a Thunder Bay prison guard to the four-year solitary confinement of a young Indigenous man named Adam Capay. Mandhane asked to see Capay and found him alone in a Plexiglas cell with no windows; the glaring artificial lights were kept on for twenty-four hours every day. His long isolation had caused memory loss, and he had trouble speaking because of the lack of human contact.[51] Public outrage resulted in Capay's release from solitary confinement and a review of segregation practices by the province. Yet in 2017, the artist Moses (Amik) Beaver of Nibinamik First Nation was found unresponsive in the same jail after prolonged struggles with mental health episodes.[52]

Through the Indian Act, the Canadian government controls nearly all health, education, and social services for Indigenous people. A 2 percent funding cap put in place in 1996 as a temporary fiscal restraint has never been lifted, even though the First Nations population has increased by more than 25 percent.[53] According to the Constitution Act of 1867, Indigenous people are a federal responsibility, and the federal government is mandated to provide health services to registered Indians living on reserve and to Inuit who live in Quebec and Labrador, explains Josée G. Lavoie of the University of Northern British Columbia. A variety of health programs and clinics funded by the federal government are on reserves, and the Non-Insured Health Benefits program provides coverage for all First Nations and Inuit people, no matter where they live.

Coverage includes dental care, drug needs, medical transport, and mental health counselling. However, the provinces are responsible for providing health and hospital care. As a result, funding comes from a patchwork of federal and provincial sources that are often difficult to access. While Indigenous political bodies are starting to gain control of federal health care funding, policy and service gaps, along with "jurisdictional ambiguity," continue to undermine progress on health care delivery and access.[54]

In 1984, the federal government adopted the Canada Health Act, which governs how funding for health care services is transferred to the provinces. Its primary objective is "to protect, promote and restore the physical and mental well-being of residents of Canada and to facilitate reasonable access to health services without financial or other barriers."[55]

But none of that is happening in Northern Ontario. When Mike Kirlew looks at the way health care is administered in the North, he sees a population of people who have been denied services from the very start. "The system isn't broken; it is designed to do what it is doing," he says.

One of his patients, an Elder, once told him, "I don't want to talk about reconciliation. I want to talk about rights." Mike couldn't agree more: "The goal of reconciliation isn't just to be friends. Civil rights legislation needs to occur here."

He believes that structurally the system — the health and social services system — is designed to fail Indigenous children. He sees children routinely taken away from their parents by social workers and shuffled from home to home to home. He knows of one small child who was moved forty-six times. "What is the fundamental mindset of doing that?" he asks. "How do you even vaccinate that child?" Time and time again, the children are taken away and the parents are left to their own devices. "I don't see bad parents," he says. "I see parents with addictions."

The medical system that operates in Canada is not structured to look at the historical systemic racism that affects Indigenous families every day. "Our mindset is that the families are deficient," he says. "But what we need to ask is 'How do we support these families and keep them together? How do we surround these children with care?'"

It is now in vogue for Canadian federal politicians to talk about how the system needs to be Indigenized, culturally adapted for First Nations, Métis, and Inuit. In April 2017, Health Canada finally agreed to cover the cost of providing an escort to the hospital for women who are about to give birth. Previously, a pregnant woman was sent alone on a plane to a city hospital, even though doctors always request that the mother have someone to assist in the labour. That practice had always been denied by the federal Indigenous health funder, the First Nations and Inuit Health Branch of Health Canada.[56] When the government announced the change and called it a great success, Mike's response was, "That is not innovative; it is just not hurting people today. Health care and education are *need*-informed care."

Mike points to the story of Brian Sinclair, an Indigenous man who died of a treatable bladder infection after waiting thirty-four hours in a Winnipeg emergency room in September 2008. Sinclair was a double amputee, confined to a wheelchair. The staff assumed he was drunk or homeless and killing time in the ER, said his cousin Robert Sinclair.[57] No one stopped to check on him, even when he vomited on himself. The inquest into Sinclair's death resulted in sixty-three recommendations, including a review of all emergency-department floor plans to ensure that patients requiring medical care are visible from the triage desk and that health authorities check that those waiting in emergency are awakened at regular intervals.[58]

"It wasn't what we saw; it was what we thought we saw that killed him," Mike says. "If you are conditioned not to care, you are conditioned to indifference. And there is a violence to that indifference." Maybe the question Canadians need to ask themselves is deeper, he says: "Why don't we care? Maybe that is the issue. Not just 'What can we do?'"

BEFORE HE WAS ELECTED as a member of provincial parliament for the Northwestern Ontario riding of Kiiwetinoong, Sol Mamakwa, a carefully spoken father of five from Kingfisher Lake First Nation, was NAN's top health advisor. He explains that the core of NAN's health transformation agenda is wresting control from the federal government and putting the power of health care into the hands of the First Nations people.

Replacing him at NAN was John Cutfeet, a former band councillor of Treaty No. 9 community Kitchenuhmaykoosib Inninuwug, who, as health transformation lead, is part of a small team (led by former National Chief of the Assembly of First

Nations Ovide Mercredi) working to change the way health care is delivered to the Nation's communities. He and his brother James Cutfeet, NAN's director of health policy and advocacy, believe that it is integral to the health of the people that they act as custodians of the land and the environment.

The difference in the quality of medical care for First Nations versus non-Indigenous people in Northern Ontario is utterly stark. There are no doctors in the NAN communities. Health or nursing stations vary in staffing levels from community to community. Some are ill-equipped, with few supplies and poorly trained staff. As a result, First Nations lack basic health care, access to medication, treatment of chronic illnesses such as diabetes, and diagnostic equipment such as X-ray machines. The provincial Ambulance Act, which requires timely dispatch of motor and air ambulance services, does not apply to reserves. Nor do the Fire Prevention and Protection Act and the Health Care Quality Act. "There are no minimum standards for anything in these environments," says Mike.

In spring 2015, the auditor general of Canada, Michael Ferguson, reported that First Nations in remote Northern Ontario and Manitoba communities did not have proper access to health care, unlike other provincial residents in small, isolated rural communities. He also found that Health Canada was not conducting regular reviews of the nursing stations.

Ferguson looked at the twenty-two federally funded nursing stations in Manitoba — twenty-one run by Health Canada nurses and one by a First Nations community — and the twenty-nine in Ontario, twenty-five operated by Health Canada nurses and four by First Nations communities.[59] "We found deficiencies in the way nursing staff and stations are managed. For example, only 1 in 45 nurses included in our sample had completed all of Health Canada's mandatory training courses," Ferguson wrote in his report.[60] These five courses cover advanced cardiac life support, pediatric advanced life support, trauma life support, immunization competencies, and the handling of controlled substances in First Nations health facilities.[61]

The auditor also found that in eight nursing stations, Health Canada had not addressed twenty-six of thirty health-and-safety or building code deficiencies. Those issues ranged from malfunctioning heating and cooling systems to unsafe stairways, ramps, and doors. In one instance, health specialists refused to visit the community because the septic tank at the residence they used had been backed up for more than two years.[62]

Nursing stations are important because they are the patient's first and only conduit to medical care. The nurses conduct assessments and decide which patients need to be flown out for further care or for appointments with therapists or specialists. Transporting patients on small chartered planes is run through a branch of Health Canada's Non-Insured Health Benefit Medical Transportation program. But NIHB clerks commonly deny NAN patients transport. In fact, the Auditor General discovered that five thousand denials of requests for medical transport from 2013 and 2014 had been investigated by Health Canada.[63]

Child health care is practically non-existent in the North. Jordan's Principle, a federal government-approved principle stating that all children should receive equitable health and social services, is barely applied in these communities. That has been the crux of Cindy Blackstock and the First Nations Child and Family Caring Society's decade-long fight against the government at the Canadian Human Rights Tribunal — to advocate for basic human rights for Indigenous children.

Children in the North are also dying of preventable diseases. Two children recently died from strep throat, and in 2014 two four-year-old children died of rheumatic fever that community care providers failed to diagnose. According to one medical study published in 2015, rheumatic fever rates are seventy-five times higher in northern First Nations communities, because of overcrowded housing and a lack of a public health care.[64]

Opioid use is rampant, and First Nations are unable to deal with the addiction epidemic. In some communities, opioid use is especially high, at 80 percent or more. Addictions counsellors are rare, and opioid substitution programs are in high demand.[65]

The availability of mental health care for children everywhere is an issue, but in Indigenous communities the situation is even worse.[66] If a child needs immediate help because of a crisis or behavioural problems, they have to be flown out to a city centre. Thunder Bay, the regional referral hospital, has only 1.2 dedicated child psychiatrists for the entire region. The 0.2 represents a psychiatrist who works part-time with children and spends the rest of her work time on research.

When it comes to suicide, the burden is almost

unbearable. The existing mental health services are barely coping with what in some communities is an acute crisis among children and youth. The Thunder Bay Regional Health Sciences Centre is the only hospital in all of Northwestern Ontario that provides in-patient psychiatric care. It is also the only institution that has staff trained to work with children fifteen years old or younger. The facility has only eight beds, and it is always at capacity. In some cases the overflow is sent to the pediatric department. For those over the age of fifteen, the other psychiatric beds are in Thunder Bay and Kenora. Both are almost always functioning over capacity.

Dr. Peter Voros, the executive vice-president of in-patient care programs, explains that children need a transitional space, a step-down unit where they can be stabilized before they are sent home. Once the children are treated there, however, there is no place to send them, so they stay in hospital. Some mentally fragile youth are sent alone to a medical facility thousands of kilometres away from their home communities.

"The only facilities that are secure are either in the south or in other provinces," Voros says. "When you send them to southern Ontario or to

British Columbia, they've got nobody. They are so disconnected."[67]

Voros says the community also needs a secure treatment facility solely for mental health and addiction patients, and ideally seven child psychiatrists to handle the patient load. He needs four to just barely function. And he needs them yesterday.

Identifying risk factors for suicidal behaviour begins with examining the age at which a person first attempts suicide. Those who try it in their teens or twenties are more likely to have "cumulative risks," such as anxiety disorders, a history of emotional and sexual abuse, or cannabis misuse.[68] If a fifteen-year-old comes from a poor, unstable household, suffers from malnourishment and abuse, is bullied at school, and suddenly receives news that a friend has died or has gone through an emotional breakup, they are at greater risk of suicide than a fifty-year-old who has just lost their job.

According to the *Saskatchewan First Nations Suicide Prevention Strategy*, in addition to suicidal triggers, a person's "developmental trajectory" needs to be examined because of the significant role that our childhoods have on how "healthy, resilient, and productive we are as youth and as adults."[69] A growing body of study shows that adverse childhood experiences impact a child's later health outcomes. The Centers for Disease Control in the United States examined the effects of sexual, physical, and emotional abuse during childhood, and of growing up "witnessing domestic violence, parental separation or divorce, and living with sub-stance-abusing, mentally ill, or criminal household members. The most damaging form of adverse childhood experiences is child sexual abuse." The CDC study concluded that 80 percent of suicide attempts during childhood and adolescence can be traced back to adverse childhood events. And these children have an increased risk of suicide over their entire lives that is "of an order of magnitude rarely observed in epidemiology and public health data."[70]

Addiction expert and BC physician Gabor Maté also points to the environment of early childhood development as a precursor to suicide:

At the core of the suicide pandemic is unresolved trauma, passed . . . from one generation to the next, along with social conditions that induce further hopelessness. The source of that mul-tigenerational trauma is this country's colonial past and its residue in the present. The march of the history and progress Canada celebrates, from which we derive much pride and national identity, meant catastrophe for natives: the loss of lands and livelihood and of freedom of movement, the mockery and invalidation of their spiritual ways, the near-extirpation of their culture, the corruption of their intrafamilial and intracommunal relationships, and finally, for nearly a hundred years, the state-sanctioned abduction, rape, physical abuse and mental torture of their children.[71]

Jack Hicks, along with his colleague Dr. Allison Crawford, director of the Northern Psychiatric Outreach Program at the Centre for Addiction and Mental Health — Canada's largest mental health teaching hospital — conducted a study comparing Indigenous communities with high incidences of youth suicide to those that have lower rates. They found that early childhood adversity may be "understood as a key mechanism by which disruption and loss related to colonization is mediated into suicidal behaviour"; as examples of colonization, they cite residential schooling and forced relocation from ancestral land.[72] The World Health Organization's 2014 report on suicide prevention came to a similar conclusion — there is a link between childhood adversity and later morbidity or mortality by means of suicide.[73]

A child born into a home affected by colonization — a home that has experienced the loss of language or connection to its cultural history, knowledge, and traditions — enters an environment marked by unresolved intergenerational trauma. Parents may be grappling with their own adverse childhood experiences, having gone through the foster system or residential school. As a result, they may suffer from mental health issues or addictions that can trigger domestic violence. Childhood adversity, Hicks and Crawford note, includes exposure to family violence; physical, emotional, and sexual abuse; neglect; and lack of access to interventions or medical care. All these factors can lead to increased risk for suicidal behaviour.[74]

"We must appreciate relevant early life risk and protective factors, and find novel and efficacious ways of intervening," Hicks and Crawford conclude. "We need to address upstream risk factors by promoting optimal early childhood development and reducing socioeconomic and early life disadvantage."[75]

But interventions have to be designed and implemented by Indigenous people and communities.

This is why early childhood development is a central part of the Inuit's 2010 Nunavut Suicide Prevention Strategy and 2016 National Inuit Suicide Prevention Strategy.[76]

The fight for social equity — for providing the basic determinants of health to Indigenous people — is not merely rhetoric. It is a matter of life or death.

DOING NOTHING IS NOT an option, yet Canada is the only G8 country without a national suicide strategy. In Scandinavia, Gunn Heatta helped establish the Sami Psychiatric Youth Team in 1990 in the small town of Karasjok, in response to a suicide cluster of young Sami men in the mid-1980s. By 2001 it had become a crucial part of the Sami National Centre on Mental Health and Substance Abuse (SANKS).[77]

Karasjok, which has a population of roughly three thousand, is nestled deep in the interior of Finnmark, near the northern Finnish border. This area, known as Inner Finnmark, is rugged terrain sprinkled with tall white birch and fir trees and fast-moving clear-water rivers. Inner Finnmark resembles in both look and feel the remote regions of Northern Ontario. Tromsø, about four hundred kilometres north of the Arctic Circle, is the only large town in the area. Brightly coloured homes are nestled among the fjords lined with white-capped mountains, and the settlement clings to the coastline. It's famous as an ideal location to see the northern lights or go whale-watching. In its heyday, many years ago, it was a centre for seal hunting, trapping, and fishing.[78] In this idyllic northern climate, the midnight sun is a constant during the summer months. The majority of people who live in Karasjok and the adjacent town of Kautokeino are Sami. There are small wooden homes belonging to the reindeer herders, and if you're lucky, you'll catch a glimpse of reindeer wandering across the road or grazing in the valley as the herds continue on their trek.

I met Gunn outside Lakselv, Norway, in a small Sami hotel north of the Arctic Circle in May of 2018. A slight, elegant woman, she has a grey bob and funky, partly horn-rimmed glasses that frame her petite face. She began her career as a therapist forty years ago, and has since felt compelled to do something to stop the suicides. SANKS officials say there are no official statistics on how many Sami have taken their lives throughout the years. That is part of their battle — trying to collect accurate numbers from health officials, which is difficult because of the national borders and differing national protocols. A social worker by training, Gunn formed a team of practitioners who fanned out, visiting schools, clubs, and other local spots to convince youth to seek counselling with Sami-trained professionals instead of turning to the traditional medical system if they or someone they knew was in crisis.

If any of the youth had suicidal thoughts or struggled with alcohol addictions, Gunn gave out her private cellphone number and told them to call her, whatever the time of day. Everyone told her she was crazy for doing that, but no one abused the privilege; she received calls only from teens in dire need of help. "I know we saved lives when people called us," Gunn says, reclining into the deep sofa. We're sitting in a log cabin in Karasjok that operates as a hotel for passing tourists.

Gunn never thought that she would still be in this position so many years later, leading the sanks team that administers mental health and addiction services for the Sami people in the Finnmark area. sanks prides itself on not being part of the Norwegian health system. Instead, its treatments

are based on Sami values and culture, are carried out in Sami language according to traditional
teachings, and include trips out onto the land to
provide youth with a holistic understanding of who
they are and where they come from.

In 2001, the Government of Norway gave
funding to SANKS to address the mental health
and substance abuse issues that were plaguing
the North. Gunn and her team formed a national
Sami competency centre and worked specifically
with people afflicted by suicidal behaviour, broken families, substance abuse, and the aftermath
of family violence.

As part of this work, the SANKS program runs
a coveted treatment centre for children and their
families, which includes one month of residential care for children and families in crisis. Entire
families are moved into one of a half-dozen IKEA-
inspired townhouses, called "apartments," on the
SANKS property. The families are not penalized
by their employers while they live at the facility,
where they receive in-patient clinical care by a staff
of trained mental health workers. The underlying
belief is that in order to treat the child or adolescent, you must also treat the parents.

The families, with children from infancy to

age eighteen, stay for four weeks. During the first week, staff get to know the family. Children attend the on-site school, and all of the meals are based on the traditional Sami diet — lots of reindeer meat and fresh salmon. In the second week, part of the treatment is a trip onto the land. Everyone goes — the entire family and its team of mental health workers. Depending on the time of year, they stay in either log cabins or in tipis, which for centuries the Sami have used when they follow the herds. The tall white canvas tipis are nearly identical to the ones the Anishinaabe use in Northern Ontario.

The program has had incredible results, but it hasn't been easy to set up or maintain. SANKS is in a constant tug-of-war with its government funders on the cost-efficiency and necessity of Indigenous-led and -created programs.

"We haven't had suicides here in the Karasjok region for several years now. But the young Sami reindeer herders in southern Sweden and Norway are now feeling it," Gunn says, referring to an increase in suicides elsewhere in Scandanavia.

IN 2007, MORE THAN five thousand distinct groups representing 370 million Indigenous people received long-overdue global recognition of their rights when 143 countries signed the United Nations Declaration on the Rights of Indigenous Peoples (UNDRIP).[79] While UNDRIP is non-binding, it should be noted that the United States, Canada, Australia, and New Zealand were the only four countries that did not initially sign it. Two years later, in 2009, Australia and New Zealand finally did sign, and the U.S. signed on in 2010, with President Barack Obama calling the declaration "one of the most significant developments in international human rights laws in decades."[80] In May 2016, Canada's minister of Indigenous affairs, Carolyn Bennett, announced in New York that Canada would no longer be the lone opposer to UNDRIP.[81]

On May 30, 2018, a private member's bill ensuring that Canadian laws conform with the principles set out in UNDRIP passed unanimously in the House of Commons. The bill was brought forward by residential school survivor Romeo Saganash, a New Democrat member of Parliament. Previously, Saganash had spent twenty-three years negotiating UNDRIP at the United Nations. "So far in this country, we haven't seen any movement towards recognizing Indigenous rights as human rights,"

Saganash said. "Our rights to clean drinking water, our rights to housing. They're not considered as human rights in this country."[82]

And without basic human rights, there will never be reconciliation.

FIVE

WE ARE NOT GOING ANYWHERE

THEY CALLED IT THE Quiet Riot.

Back in March 1987, Rance Christianson, from Kingfisher Lake First Nation, was a seventeen-year-old grade eleven student at Stirland Lake, a Mennonite-run Indian Residential School in Northern Ontario.

While most residential schools closed in the 1960s and 1970s, the Mennonite Church began to establish its own residential schools in the North, starting in the late 1950s.[1] Stirland Lake, also known as Wahbon Bay Academy, opened its doors in 1971, 273 kilometres north of Sioux Lookout in the deep, dense boreal forest. The school, made up of old buildings delivered by flatbed truck from a mine at Pickle Crow, had become coeducational after the school for girls, Cristal Lake, closed in 1986.[2]

Rance remembers how strict the instructors were at Stirland and how the school felt more like a prison than the one he had attended in Winnipeg for grades nine and ten. The students were not allowed to listen to rock music, which the teachers called "devil's music." Cassette tapes of bands like Mötley Crüe and the Rolling Stones were confiscated. The students could listen only to Mennonite hymns. Their mail was censored so they couldn't tell their parents what was happening inside those school walls.

"We couldn't write a bad thing about what we were experiencing. And if we did something they didn't like, they would give us demerit points. Sometimes we'd have to go out in the winter and saw hundreds of logs with a handsaw," he recalls.[3] The winters north of Sioux Lookout can dip to temperatures around minus forty. "They wanted us to be robots, under control. 'You do this' or 'you do that.' Not realizing that when you are out there and isolated and held down by rigid rules, you want your freedom."

The boys lived in dorms, separate from the girls. By 10:30 p.m., it was lights out. The students had to be at breakfast at seven sharp every morning, and if they were late they had to do chores. The food, Rance remembers, was "really crappy, and only on Sundays were there home-cooked meals." For breakfast, they were always served greasy oats with goat's milk. Saturday mornings were special — they had cornflakes.

The teachers used corporal punishment to keep the students in line. Normally, such disciplinary action came out of nowhere. Suddenly a pupil was picked out of a class or a hallway and they were brutally bullied and made an example of.

Rance remembers what they did to him as if it were yesterday. "They called us, one by one, to a certain dormitory and took us downstairs. There were four adult men waiting down there. Two of them held my arms and legs, and one put his whole body weight on me while the other strapped me with a paddle, really hard. He caused a lot of bruising. By the time he was done, I was in agony; [it was] torture."

When they were finished, they got the scissors out and cut his hair. He felt violated all over again. "In my case, they just didn't strap me; to humiliate me further, they cut off my hair. "

Rance never received any medical treatment. For

a week, his behind was black, bruised all over. He could walk, but sitting down was excruciating, and when the bruising began to heal, it itched something awful.

"They did it to all of us. They took great enjoyment out of it. It was sadistic. It was far away from their religious upbringing," he says. "For all the good things you hear about Mennonites, this was not the case with these guys. I don't know, this was like prison or something. They ran a prison school."

After his beating, Rance and the other, older students began to talk. They had to do something. They eventually decided that if the teachers tried to hit another student, they were going to resist.

Then, one evening, when some of the male students met some of the females past curfew, the teachers struck. They caught one of the teen boys; another ran off to tell Rance.

"I said, 'Okay, that is enough.' I grabbed a stick, and about five of us went out there to go challenge our abusers," he says. They confronted the teachers on the roadside. "As we challenged them, we started engaging physically with them, hitting them, fighting them, and they were fighting back and then they started retreating."

Their abusers fell back into one of the dorms.

But the students were not done. They busted the windows and trashed the other buildings.

"That is what we did, in retaliation for what they did," he says.

For one night, it seemed the students had won. They had succeeded in standing up to their tormentors, and they were finally in control. Until morning light came.

"They sent the police in the morning after, and the police came in with assault rifles, shotguns, whatever. Basically, we were unarmed. But they came in to restore order," Rance says. "A few of us got arrested and taken away to Pickle Lake. There was no plan for us to return home. Some of us were just arrested with the shirts on our backs, no proper clothing."

The boys had to make court appearances. From the start, they were treated as criminals.

"Many of us were charged for the first time. We didn't know how to defend ourselves. So we all got charged with mischief, riot, assault, different charges under the Young Offenders Act," Rance remembers. "I recall the same bunch, the same people, were just smirking at us. They weren't good people. They were evil people."

Rance lost his school year and had to repeat

grade eleven in Marathon, Ontario. Some of his classmates have since passed away, including one friend from North Spirit Lake who died by suicide. Rance understands the drinking, the drugs, the destroyed spirit after residential school. The anger and pain manifest in different ways for different people. Life at Stirland, he says, "was mockery of our human dignity. That is what it was."

The Stirland Lake Quiet Riot is not written up in any news reports or in any history books. But it was part of a movement that traces back to the civil rights era in the United States.

"I think our riot was the first of its kind [at a residential school] to enable us to stand up for our rights as people. We were fighting against a colonization system. We were fighting against colonization."

He knows the fight isn't over.

THE STRONG, LOUD PULSE of the drum beat in perfect time, like the steady thumping of the human heart, and it filled the lobby of the Delta Hotel in downtown Ottawa, on the unceded territory of the Algonquins, whose land the Parliament of Canada sits on. It is unceded because this land was not surrendered or given away. It is still the subject of treaty negotiations with the Government of Canada, the Province of Ontario, and the Crown.

On May 23, 2018, a First Nations–led conference called determinATION: Moving Beyond the Indian Act was about to begin. The airy, light-filled lobby smelled of sweet smoke. A smudge ceremony was taking place in the grand ballroom, where First Nations and Métis were meeting. The conference, organized by the grand chief of the Nishnawbe Aski Nation, Alvin Fiddler, brought together an impressive list of close to three hundred First Nations Elders, leaders, knowledge keepers, youth, and lawyers for two days at the Delta to imagine a future without the Indian Act. All the progressives, all the thinkers, were there: lawyer Bev Jacobs, one of the first presidents of the Native Women's Association of Canada; Ovide Mercredi, former national chief of the Assembly of First Nations; youth leader Max FineDay; and a number of grand chiefs representing British Columbia and the far reaches of Ontario. Co-hosting the conference was Osgoode Hall Law School.

On July 14, 2017, the elected government of Prime Minister Justin Trudeau had promised a renewal of Canada's relationship with Indigenous Peoples, one that would eventually lead to dismantling of the

Indian Act.[4] Through its "engagement process," the government aimed to develop a framework recognizing Indigenous rights as stated in Section 35 of the 1982 Constitution Act. Section 35 recognizes and affirms existing rights, but it does not define them — so Canada's courts have taken up much of that task.[5]

Trudeau maintained that if Indigenous communities could define Section 35, they would be in charge of their own destinies. Jody Wilson-Raybould, Canada's first Indigenous attorney general and current minister of justice, confirmed that this would be a major step towards self-determination and self-government. For the first time in Canadian history, First Nations would be able to define their own "full box of rights," based on what was good for their own communities, thus putting them in control of land rights, education policy, and child welfare.[6] "This is a marriage, not a divorce," said Indigenous Services Minister Carolyn Bennett.[7]

The night before the summit began, Alvin and I went for dinner with Mushkegowuk Grand Council Chief Jonathan Solomon at a chain steakhouse restaurant across the street from the hotel. The place was packed with Indigenous people from across the country. We sat down in a small booth and Alvin asked Jonathan how his news conference had gone. Earlier that day, at the National Press Theatre, Jonathan and New Democratic MP Charlie Angus had stood before the TV cameras to call for a national suicide strategy.

Jonathan and his people have taken a leadership role in addressing this issue. As part of their People's Inquiry, four commissioners travelled up and down Ontario's James Bay coast, holding public hearings, and seventy-seven individual stories were collected. The stories were published "so that others will understand the causes and the profound impacts of suicide in our communities. We share them so that others can learn from listening to the storytellers' experiences. We share them to break the silence, and to encourage our people to continue to speak openly, while respecting and supporting one another. We share their suggestions, because we believe the solutions lie within us."[8]

At the conclusion of their work, they identified sixteen key issues — top among them the Indian Residential School experience, sexual abuse, substance abuse, lack of parenting skills, and a loss of identity and culture. Each of the issues came with a set of solutions, from programs that reintroduce youth to the land through guided field trips — like Ed Metatawabin's expedition down the Albany River, and another with teens from Kashechewan First Nation who paddle more than four hundred kilometres down the Albany — to securing funding from government, resource companies, and institutions; to promoting healing from and awareness of sexual abuse.

Jonathan's communities had been among the hardest hit by suicide. Attawapiskat made international headlines in April 2017. Before that, in late 2013, Attawapiskat Chief Theresa Spence held a six-week-long fast on Victoria Island, just a stone's throw from Parliament Hill, to protest the community's living conditions and to demand a meeting with Prime Minister Stephen Harper to discuss Indigenous rights.[9]

In January 2017, Jonathan had gone to Ottawa with Alvin and Wapekeka First Nation's band manager, Joshua Frogg, to hold a press conference after the two twelve-year-old girls from Wapekeka, one of whom was Frogg's niece, died by suicide. Jonathan and Joshua called attention to the federal government's failure to acknowledge the community's plea for assistance, despite having been warned of the suicide pact.[10] Ultimately, seven girls from

Wapekeka and Poplar Hill First Nation who knew each other took their lives.

One year later, Jonathan was still calling on the government for aid. "There have been numerous calls to action on this sad and tragic issue. There have been reactionary measures announced. But I am here with my colleagues and professionals to call on the prime minister and the Government of Canada to begin discussions on a national strategy on suicide prevention . . . We don't need another study or inquiry. Everything has been studied and these studies are just collecting dust on a shelf," he told the TV cameras.[11]

Shortly after the deaths of the twelve-year-old girls from Wapekeka, Canadian Prime Minister Justin Trudeau had asked Jonathan, Joshua, and Alvin for a private meeting to discuss what could be done to prevent more of their children from dying by suicide.

"It was there that I challenged the prime minister that he could be a champion to lead a national strategy on suicide prevention and intervention," Jonathan said. "His government has passed two national budgets since then and I am still waiting."[12]

Everyone at the determinATION conference was in agreement — Indigenous self-governance must not be dictated by the Indian Act. Communities and Nations should no longer be forced to abandon their culture and spiritual practices, assimilate into the dominant society, adhere to federal governance of reserves, and have to register to be considered real Indians by law in order to receive their treaty rights. Communities and Nations must be empowered to design their own path forward.

NAN Grand Chief Alvin Fiddler walked up to the podium to give the opening address. The 1929 adhesion to Treaty No. 9 — at the signing of which Alvin's father, Moses, was present — expanded Crown territory to include Kitchenuhmaykoosib Inninuwug and communities along the Windigo, Fort Severn, and Winisk Rivers. But Alvin believes that First Nations people did not surrender jurisdiction over their land.

Alvin has been at the helm of change for his people in Northern Ontario. He led the push for the joint inquest looking into the circumstances around the deaths of the seven NAN youth attending high school in Thunder Bay, and he served on the Truth and Reconciliation Commission as manager of regional and Ontario liaisons, in charge of collecting the testimony of survivors of one of the darkest chapters in Canadian history — the

residential school era, which decimated generations of Indigenous families and has subsequently
led to mass incarceration of Indigenous people; a
child welfare system that routinely separates First
Nations children from their families and home
communities and places them in state care; addictions and self-medication to deal with the trauma,
abuse, and displacement; and a youth suicide rate
that is five to seven times higher than that of the
non-Indigenous youth population.[13]

Alvin is taking steps to decolonize the health
system in Northern Ontario. On November 17,
2017, he signed the Joint Action Table Health
Transformation Work Plan with the federal and
provincial governments to develop a community-
driven system with adequate funding to better
serve the forty-nine First Nations that make up
NAN. For the first time in 150 years, the First
Nations in Northern Ontario will be in full control of their health care.

"Our communities are in a perpetual state of
crisis, and health transformation is the pathway
to improving outcomes for our people. This is a
monumental undertaking, but we are confident that
by working together with leaders, policy-makers,
health care administrators and providers we can

build a health system that works for our people," Alvin said at the time of the signing.[14]

In his opening statement at determiNATION, Alvin told a quiet audience that he no longer wanted to be identified by a ten-digit number given to him by the federal government. "I took my card out the other day, looked at it, and realized it had expired about four years ago," he said. "That must mean I am an expired Indian."

The audience laughed.

He continued to talk about the current imperative — that another generation of First Nations children not have to grow up under the shadow of the Indian Act. As a father of two daughters, he wants to live to see the day when their existence is no longer legitimized by assigned numbers or dictated by the federal government, effectively making them wards of the state.

Alvin believes it is not up to the government to determine who is Indigenous and who is not.

Belonging is not theirs to give.

HISTORY IS SHARED; NOTHING happens in isolation.

The violent colonization of the Americas paved the way for the extermination of Native Americans and the enslavement of African Americans in the United States, which has led to the clash between the races that we see now. In his 1964 book *Why We Can't Wait*, Martin Luther King Jr. identified the struggle of Black people in the United States with the history of the Native Americans:

> Our nation was born in genocide when it embraced the doctrine that the original American, the Indian, was an inferior race. Even before there were large numbers of Negroes on our shores, the scar of racial hatred had already disfigured colonial society. From the sixteenth century forward, blood flowed in battles of racial supremacy. We are perhaps the only nation which has tried as a matter of national policy to wipe out its Indigenous population. Moreover, we elevated that tragic experience into a noble crusade. Indeed, even today we have not permitted ourselves to reject or feel remorse for this shameful episode. Our literature, our films, our drama, our folklore all exalt it.[15]

King's formidable presence, along with the Black Power movement, which came out of the civil rights struggle, influenced a generation of Native

American activists. In 1968, the American Indian Movement (AIM) was founded by Chippewa activists Dennis Banks, Clyde Bellecourt, Eddie Benton Banai, and George Mitchell in Minneapolis, Minnesota.[16] AIM fought for social justice and economic progress for Native Americans and protested unlawful arrests by organizing neighbourhood patrols to monitor police activities.[17]

From November 20, 1969, to June 11, 1971, members of AIM helped stage a takeover of Alcatraz Island. Eighty-nine Native Americans, under the title Indians of All Tribes, came together to occupy the prison island in a symbolic reclamation of abandoned and out-of-use federal lands, as was agreed upon under the terms of the 1868 Treaty of Fort Laramie with the Sioux Nation.[18] During that nineteen-month period, Native American delegations from all over the world visited the island, offering provisions and support to the protestors.[19]

Members of AIM also came up to Kenora, Northwestern Ontario, in the summer of 1974 to add their support in the armed occupation of what is now Anicinabe Park, a traditional gathering place for Ojibwe. Louie Cameron, a founder of the Ojibway Warriors Society (OWS), had organized a conference in the park to discuss long-standing local issues and frustrations, such as a lack of access to health care, poor living conditions, and over-policing. Cameron was from nearby Wabaseemoong First Nation. Also at the top of everyone's minds was the fact that the Government of Canada had sold the land to the City of Kenora in 1959 without the consent of the Ojibwe.[20] The meeting erupted with anger and the 150 OWS members in attendance staged an occupation, which lasted thirty-nine days.

"This was the youth's idea. They were determined," recalls Richard Green, from Shoal Lake 40 First Nation, who was a good friend of Cameron's. "They weren't taking it anymore. We have a face, a culture, a people. There was an awakening."[21]

The Indians of All Tribes Occupation of Alcatraz Island thrust Native American activism into the nation's consciousness, effectively inspiring other young Native Americans, including John Echohawk, who in 1970 founded and became the executive director of the Native American Rights Fund (NARF). Echohawk based NARF on the NAACP's Legal Defense and Education Fund, having been inspired by Dr. King's words about equality and self-determination and the right to live as tribes under the tribal sovereignty laws that were first created in 1831.[22] The non-profit legal firm works to protect the status, sovereignty, and treaty rights of tribes.[23] Among NARF's many projects is representation of the Rosebud Sioux Tribe in protesting the Keystone XL pipeline, which cuts through the Lakota Nation's Nebraska homelands. NARF has also worked with the Standing Rock Sioux Tribe lawyers in order to mount a strong, united legal strategy before the U.S. federal courts.[24]

The Standing Rock Sioux Tribe and First Nations and allies from across Turtle Island came together to protest the construction of the 1,172-mile Dakota Access Pipeline, which would carry over half a million barrels of Bakken crude oil across four states.[25] The Sioux say they were not adequately consulted about construction of the pipeline, which would cross Lake Oahe, half a mile from Standing Rock's reserve, thus damaging sacred sites, contaminating drinking water, and violating the Nation's treaty rights.

In April 2016, a historic gathering of Indigenous Nations took place at the Oceti Sakowin Camp, near Cannon Ball, North Dakota.[26] The Sioux Elders foretold of the coming of the "black snake" that must be stopped in order to safeguard the water of life, to keep it *Mni Woc'oni*, pure and sacred.[27] Those who came brought their own tents, tipis, and supplies and braved the harsh conditions on the plains. At one point, thousands were marching daily and holding ceremonies.

In early September 2016, a small delegation from Nishnawbe Aski Nation — Travis Boissoneau, Derek Fox, Mike McKay, Sol Mamakwa, and Bill Maloney — arrived at the Oceti Sakowin Camp. They were carrying the NAN flag, the central emblem of which is the white bear, symbolizing the strength, unity, and community of the forty-nine Northern First Nations. They placed their flag alongside all the other flags representing Indigenous Nations from across North America. The group walked with the protectors, chanting, "Clean water for your children and grandchildren!" For them, this was not just about clean water for Indigenous people — this was about clean water for all. The protectors clashed with the pipeline's security guards, who stood in a line along the road, holding tight the leashes of their snarling dogs. "I could not believe what was happening," says Sol, who is a Stirland Lake Residential School survivor.

By February 2017, a new president was in the White House. One of Donald Trump's first orders was to resume construction of the pipeline. By the end of February, what was left of the Standing

Rock camps was brought down and the people were evicted. By April 2017, the pipeline was completed.

Still, the significance of Standing Rock cannot be underestimated. It was the first time that so many Indigenous Nations from across the continent stood together in a peaceful protest. This is the victory of Standing Rock. Unity.

There are connections between all of these liberation struggles. There is a connection between Standing Rock and the Occupation of Alcatraz and Idle No More, which has become one of the largest Indigenous rights movements in Canadian history. That campaign was started by three First Nations women and one ally in November 2012, in protest of Bill c-45, legislation that would allow federal and provincial governments and big corporations to advance large projects without environmental assessments.[28] Idle No More stands for Indigenous sovereignty, and it has prompted teach-ins, round dances, and demonstrations across Canada.

There is a connection between Idle No More and the Justice for Our Stolen Children Camp, which set up tipis in Regina in response to the acquittal of white farmer Gerald Stanley in February 2018 in the death of twenty-two-year-old Colten Boushie, a Cree man whom Stanley shot in the head, and the acquittal of Raymond Cormier in the death of fifteen-year-old Tina Fontaine, a Sagkeeng First Nation girl whose body was pulled out of Winnipeg's Red River on August 17, 2014. The camp was set up to protest the racism built into the child welfare and justice systems, which kills Indigenous men, women, Two-Spirit people, and kids every day.[29]

There is a connection between the Sami's thirteen-year fight, from 1970 to 1983, against construction of the ecologically damaging Alta Dam,[30] and Camp Cloud, the First Nations–led protest established in November 2017 against Kinder Morgan's Trans Mountain Pipeline expansion through Burnaby Mountain, British Columbia.

And there is a connection between the harmful policies and laws in all colonized nations and the present-day treatment of Indigenous Peoples in Brazil, who continue to clash with farmers, prospectors, and multinational corporations to regain ancestral land promised to them for decades by various government administrations. In February 2017, the president of Brazil, Michel Temer, proposed legislation that would, in fact, lift the limits on foreign ownership of farmland in the northern Amazon, which would effectively allow multinational corporations to buy the land, rip out the trees, and reap the profits at the expense of the Indigenous communities.[31]

There is a connection between all of these movements and the scores of others that have taken place in countries around the world for centuries, and continue to take place today.

And there is a connection to all of us.

SO, IN THIS TIME AND AGE, how does one address the seeming contradiction between progress and regression? Angela Davis, an African-American political activist and professor emerita at the University of California, poses this question in her book *Freedom Is a Constant Struggle*.[32] Davis herself was imprisoned for a time, and she credits the international efforts of rights organizations around the world with helping to free her.

"I don't really believe there is any one country whose Indigenous people are doing any better than anyone else," Dr. Helen Milroy says.[33] Helen has noticed that among the countries she has travelled to with the Wharerātā Group, an international organization of Indigenous mental health and addiction leaders from Canada, the United States, Australia,

New Zealand, Norway, and Sweden, advancements in Indigenous rights vary from country to country.

"They are more advanced in some places and going backwards in other places. Some are making greatest strides here, and others are stuck elsewhere. We don't have a parliament [in Australia], but we have a lot more development in policies and programs than the Sami. People often look to New Zealand as a shining hope, but in some respects they have gone backwards. I just think it is a struggle everywhere. In some respects, having a united voice is quite nice. You sit and learn from each other, and you are together for some of the struggle. There is such effort going on internationally, and so much commonality. Despite all of the differences we also have in our histories." She pauses and then adds: "You have to gather your allies."

In Canada, it has been more than a decade since Jordan River Anderson's father, Ernest Anderson, stood with his daughter Jermaine and witnessed Parliament vote unanimously to support Jordan's Principle, which would ensure that First Nations kids received full public services without discrimination. On February 2, 2005, five-year-old Jordan, who was born with complex disabilities known as Carey Fineman Ziter syndrome, died after spending his entire life in hospital because of a jurisdictional dispute between the federal and provincial governments on the payment of his medical bills.[34]

"Don't let the good being done in my son's name today just be a moral victory," Ernest Anderson said to Cindy Blackstock, director of the First Nations Child and Family Caring Society.[35] Blackstock took Ernest's words to heart. Since then, she has tirelessly and relentlessly fought for the equitable treatment of all Indigenous children in this country. "What I am looking for is full compliance with Jordan's Principle," Blackstock says.[36]

Still, in January 2016, the Canadian Human Rights Tribunal (CHRT) — an independent human rights commission created by the federal government — ordered Canada once again to fully implement Jordan's Principle as a matter of law. Altogether there have been four non-compliance orders.[37] The third one was issued in May 2017, following the suicides of the two girls in Wapekeka First Nation. The tribunal noted that after Wapekeka asked for help in July 2016, none came: "While Canada provided assistance once the Wapekeka suicides occurred, the flaws in the Jordan's Principle process left any chance of preventing the Wapekeka tragedy unaddressed and the tragic events only triggered a reactive response to then provide services."[38]

Even though a series of non-compliance orders has been issued, the CHRT is not without hope. In the fourth CHRT ruling, on February 1, 2018, tribunal chair Sophie Marchildon and member Edward Lustig wrote:

> It is important to look at this case in terms of bringing Justice and not simply the Law, especially with reconciliation as a goal. This country needs healing and reconciliation and the starting point is the children and respecting their rights. If this is not understood in a meaningful way, in the sense that it leads to real and measurable change, then the TRC and this Panel's work is trivialized and unfortunately the suffering is borne by vulnerable children.[39]

The panel also pointed out that Canada is working towards change. "The Panel also trusts that change has started and has accelerated in the last few months. The Panel is really hopeful for what is coming ahead for Indigenous children in Canada."[40]

Blackstock noted that while Health Canada had improved service since May 2016, the Department of Indigenous and Northern Affairs continued to abrogate its responsibilities for early childhood education and child welfare. "Kids are going into care unnecessarily as we speak," she said.

To every single one of the CHRT hearings, Blackstock brought a white teddy bear given to her by Mary Teegee of Carrier Sekani Family Services in Prince George, BC — Spirit Bear, who acts as a symbolic reminder for all in attendance to always keep the focus on the children and not the politics.[41] Keeping that in mind, the First Nations Child and Family Caring Society developed the Spirit Bear Plan, which asks all MPs to request that the parliamentary budget officer cost out the current shortfalls in all federally funded services, such as education, health care, child welfare, and clean water delivery, and come up with solutions to fix the deficiencies, in consultation with First Nations. The plan also asks for the creation of tangible target dates and short time frames for specific investments, and that all government departments do a complete analysis of services provided to Indigenous kids in order to ensure that there are no ongoing discriminatory policies or practices. It also insists that senior government workers be properly trained, as was outlined in the

Truth and Reconciliation Commission's *94 Calls to Action.*

"Let's get this behind us," Blackstock says. "Let's raise a generation of First Nations kids, for the first time in the history of this country, that actually gets the same level of services that every other kid enjoys. Children only get one childhood. Fix it today so we don't have to apologize to the next generation."[42]

WHAT IS TRUTH, and what is reconciliation?

Senator Murray Sinclair, one of the most fair-minded and respected Indigenous thinkers, believes that the education system has played a dominant role in damaging relations between First Peoples and the greater society. For generations the education system has perpetuated an ignorance and unawareness among much of society, having left conspicuously absent the other side of history, from early European colonization to the 150,000 First Nations, Métis, and Inuit children who were sent to residential schools here in Canada, and the thousands of other children who went to such schools in the United States and Norway, and to the Aborigine mission schools in Australia.

While assimilation through education did not work, the legacy of those schools is still very much present today. Those experiences live on in the minds and the nightmares of the survivors, who develop derogatory attitudes about themselves that are only reinforced by their engagement with the greater society.[43] The after-effects live on in their children, who may grow up with parents who have little knowledge of how to raise kids, and who cannot pass on their cultural traditions and languages, having been alienated from their ancestral heritage themselves. And the after-effects live on in their children's children, creating a heartbreaking legacy of family instability.

The state education system has purposefully kept the general population ignorant of the physical, cultural, and spiritual genocide Indigenous Peoples have endured for centuries. As Senator Sinclair says, "Nation-building has been the main theme of Canada's history curricula for a long time and Aboriginal people, except for a few notable exceptions trotted out as if to prove the rule, have been portrayed as bystanders, if not obstacles, to the enterprise of nation-building."[44]

Senator Sinclair was raised by his grandmother, who lovingly scrimped and saved to send him to university, and he vividly remembers sitting in a classroom and being taught that "my people were irrelevant. By implication it caused me to feel that I was too. It taught us to believe in the inferiority of Aboriginal people and in the inherent superiority of white European civilization."[45] And to get the grades he needed, he was compelled to learn this mantra instead of learning about the humanity, pride, and accomplishments of the First Peoples — their proud cultures and histories, and their advanced civilizations before the arrival of the explorer and settler nations.

He also points out that, by extension, the lawmakers, the judges, the politicians, the deep thinkers of modern Western society all grew up without the benefit of knowing the true history of their countries. So their understanding — which shaped the policies, rules, and programs of democratic nations — was flawed from the start. As a result, non-Indigenous people have struggled to understand the calls for justice and equity by leaders of these Nations. Some ask why Indigenous Peoples can't seem to get over history. And too many were taught to look away.

While education has played a huge role in damaging relations between the Indigenous and non-Indigenous communities, it is also going to play a crucial role in reconciling that relationship. In Canada, legions of teachers have taken it upon themselves to learn more about this country's true history by reading and teaching books by Indigenous authors and historians, even if their governments are not keeping pace with what they are doing in the classroom. The educators always lead us forward.

For leaders like Natan Obed, reconciliation feels far off, a distant ideal that is still out of reach. "Reconciliation takes action. It means ending social inequity," he says. "Why is it in Inuit Nunangat, the median income is $17,700 and for non-Inuit who live in Inuit Nunnagut it is $77,000? Why is it okay for us to have 250 times the rate for TB than all other Canadians born in Canada? Why is it okay that we have 40 percent overcrowding in our housing? Why is it okay that 29 percent of our adults have a high school education? These are not okay. In times of reconciliation, it is time to build a Canada for all of us and it goes beyond sympathy," he says.[46]

But what is happening in his home of Nunavut offers a glimmer of hope. The government has created the Quality of Life Secretariat within the

Department of Health to lead suicide prevention initiatives. Over five years, the Government of Nunavut is investing $35 million in programs as part of its 2017–22 Inuusivut Anninaqtuq Action Plan. Working in partnership with the government are the RCMP and the Embrace Life Council, a non-profit suicide prevention organization. The $35 million will fund community-led plans and mobile Inuktut counselling services for Arctic communities, as well as research, gatherings, and training.[47]

A large part of the strategy is to hire Inuit staff. But work in suicide prevention is not easy. Many have their own mental health issues caused by family or community trauma or as a result of bullying in previous workplaces. As a result, these individuals require coaching, support, and flexible hours to prevent them from becoming suicidal themselves.

The efforts of the Quality of Life Secretariat have resulted in the "de-normalization" of suicide. Before, it was as if no one talked about suicide, suicide attempts, or mental illness and addictions; they were simply accepted as a part of everyday life. Now they do talk about these issues more openly, which could lead to an increasing number of people's accessing treatment.

The Government of Nunavut has acknowledged that in order to stop the suicide crisis, all inequality issues must be addressed at once. Its strategy also supports reducing overcrowding, poverty, and crime. Ending social inequity extends to the justice system. At the moment, Indigenous and Black people are overrepresented in correctional facilities across Turtle Island.

In Canada, the Indigenous incarceration rates are stunning. In the 1950s and 1960s, before the Sixties Scoop and the institution of child welfare policies, about 2 percent of the prison population was Indigenous.[48] In 2018, Statistics Canada reported that Indigenous people make up about 4.1 percent of the country's population overall, but in 2016–17, Indigenous people accounted for 28 percent of admissions into the prison population in the provinces and territories, and 27 percent in federal penitentiaries. And that proportion has grown — ten years ago, it was 21 percent for the provinces and territories and 19 percent for the federal prison system.[49]

Systemic justice issues extend to bail policies, mandatory minimum penalties, and "administration of justice" offences such as not appearing in court or disobeying a court order. Many call for

Indigenous laws and traditions and restorative justice to be built into the current system.

It is clear that Indigenous Nations must be given the political and moral authority over their own communities that historically they have been denied. The current system, introduced shortly after First Contact and reinforced over the subsequent centuries, has failed. The results of that failure have been laid out in these chapters. Again I give you the words of Martin Luther King Jr.: "Justice is indivisible. Injustice anywhere is a threat to justice everywhere."[50]

We know this history of injustice to be true, yet how many times will I have to speak to a mother in North Caribou Lake or Iqaluit or Lac La Ronge about the life of a child they have just lost to suicide?

How many times will I have to hear the cracking voice of Alvin Fiddler on a small charter flight to yet another funeral of another child in a grieving community?

How many times will I see a message flash across my phone in the middle of the night that says, "Something is happening down by the river. Police lights are everywhere and they think they have found him."

How many times will I hear that a person tried

for shooting an unarmed Indigenous man to death has walked free?

Or how many times will I stand over a spot where the remains of one of our more than 1,200 murdered and missing Indigenous women and girls have been found, out on the rocks, or in the middle of the road, or at the river's edge?

Throughout these chapters, I have talked about the rights of Indigenous children, here at home and all over the world. I have talked about the determinants of health — clean water, a proper education, nutritious food, safe housing, safe communities where kids are cared for and tucked into bed by their parents. But this is not just about civil rights. This is about freedom.

I have written about the continuous genocide against the Guarani in Brazil; about the impact of the loss of their traditional way of life on the Sami in Norway, Sweden, Finland, and Russia, and Inuit in the Northern territories in Canada; about the policies of extermination in the United States; and about the decades of legislated racism against Aboriginals and Torres Strait Islanders in Australia.

I have referred to the fact that apartheid in South Africa was modelled in part on Canada's Indian Act. Nelson Mandela devoted his life to ending apartheid. But his struggle went beyond South Africa. Mandela's political emergence occurred within the context of internationalism, a coming together of people from all over the world who fought for his release from prison and the freedom of the nearly twenty million Black South Africans from an oppressive system — from Artists United Against Apartheid, led by activists Steven Van Zandt and Arthur Baker, which in 1985 released a song called "Sun City" to raise awareness of apartheid in South Africa; to artists such as Lou Reed and Bono, who refused to sing at an all-white resort; to the students on college campuses across Europe and North America who mounted scores of protests. Mandela would not want to be singled out for dismantling apartheid — it was done by legions, within South Africa and around the world.[51] As he famously said, "To be free is not merely to cast off one's chains, but to live in a way that respects and enhances the freedom of others."[52]

In a speech marking the centenary of Mandela's birth on July 18, 2018, Barack Obama paid tribute to the freedom fighter, who "came to embody the universal aspirations of dispossessed people all around the world, their hopes for a better life, the possibility for a moral transformation in the conduct of human affairs."[53]

Nations are made stronger by vibrant, healthy children. As Senator Sinclair says, "In order for any society to function properly and to its full capacity, it must raise and educate its children so that they can answer what philosophers such as Socrates, and Plato, and our Elders, call 'the great questions of life.'"[54]

Those four questions were laid out at the beginning of this book: Where do I come from? Where am I going? Why am I here? Who am I?

All children, regardless of their racial or socioeconomic backgrounds, need to know the answers to these questions. They need to know who their ancestors are, who their heroes and villains are; they need to know about their family's traditions and cultures and the community they are a part of. Our children must feel that they are loved, valued, and worthy members of society who belong in this world exactly as they are.

As Thomas King said, "But don't say in the years to come that you would have lived your life differently if only you had heard this story. You've heard it now."[55]

Aaniin. Boozhoo.
Tanya Talaga Ndishinikaaz.
Aaniin ezhinikaazoyan?
Aandi wenjibaayan?

This is where we are from.
We have always been here.
Chi-miigwech.[56]

NOTES

EPIGRAPHS

Mushkegowuk Council, *The People's Inquiry into Our Suicide Pandemic*, written and submitted October 27, 2014, published 2016, http://caid. ca/MusCouInq2016_Rep.pdf.

Thomas King, *The Truth About Stories* (Toronto: House of Anansi Press, 2003), 29, 60, 89, 119, 151, 167.

CHAPTER 1: WE WERE ALWAYS HERE

1. Interview with Beacon Home's Esther Aiken, April 2018.

2. Nishnawbe Aski Nation (website), "About Us," http://www.nan.on. ca/article/about-us-3.asp.

3. "Update from Wapekaka First Nation" (press release), Wapekeka First Nation, January 18, 2017, http://www.nan.on.ca/upload/ documents/wapekeka-press-release-jan19-2017final.pdf.

4. Interview with Anna Betty Achneepineskum, April 16, 2018.

5. Grand Chief Alvin Fiddler, letter to Prime Minister Justin Trudeau, January 18, 2017, http://www.nan.on.ca/upload/documents/letter-to-prime-minister-justin-trudeau-.pdf.

6. Jody Porter and John Paul Tasker, "Wapekeka First Nation Asked for Suicide-Prevention Funds Months before Deaths of 2 Girls," CBC News, January 19, 2017, https://www.cbc.ca/news/canada/thunder-bay/wapekeka-suicides-health-canada-1.3941439.

7. Fiddler letter to Trudeau, January 18, 2017, and Wapekeka First Nation letter, July 18, 2016, http://www.nan.on.ca/upload/documents/letter-and-proposal-from-wfn-july-18-201.pdf.

8. Mushkegowuk Council, *The People's Inquiry into Our Suicide Pandemic*, written and submitted October 27, 2014, published 2016, http://caid.ca/MusCouInq2016_Rep.pdf.

9. "NAN Welcomes Ontario's Commitment to Health Transformation as Inquest Highlights Issues" (press release), Nishnawbe Aski Nation, February 14, 2018, http://www.nan.on.ca/article/february-14-2018-22548.asp.

10. Gloria Galloway, "The System Failed My Son," *Globe and Mail*, August 19, 2015, https://www.theglobeandmail.com/news/national/first-nations-health-care-the-system-failed-myson/article26020926/.

11. "Election 2015: Closing the Aboriginal Health Gap," *Canadian Medical Association Journal*, (press release; early draft), October 5, 2015, http://www.cmaj.ca/content/cmaj/early/2015/10/05/cmaj.109-5155.full.pdf.

12. Office of the Chief Coroner (Ontario), Verdict of Coroner's Jury: Seven First Nation Youths, June 28, 2016, https://www.mcscs.jus.gov.on.ca/english/Deathinvestigations/Inquests/Verdictsandrecommendations/OCCVerdictsSevenFirstNationsYouths.html#General.

13. Susana Mas, "Trudeau Lays Out Plan for New Relationship with Indigenous People," CBC News, December 8, 2015, https://www.cbc.ca/news/politics/justin-trudeau-afn-indigenous-aboriginal-people-1.3354747.

14. Fiddler letter to Trudeau, January 18, 2017.

15. Nishnawbe Aski Nation, *Completed Suicides, 1986 to January 17, 2018* (table).

16. Centre for Suicide Prevention (website), "Indigenous Suicide Prevention," https://www.suicideinfo.ca/resource/indigenous-suicide-prevention/.

17. Testimony of Jack Hicks, House of Commons, Standing Committee on Indigenous and Northern Affairs, Evidence (Meeting no. 18, June 7, 2016), 42nd Parliament, 1st session, http://www.ourcommons.ca/DocumentViewer/en/42-1/INAN/meeting-18/evidence.

18. "In a Land of Thundering Reindeer, Suicide Stalks the Indigenous Sami," PBS, December 11, 2016, https://www.pbs.org/newshour/world/sami-indigenous-reindeer-suicide.

19. Eliza Racine, "Native Americans Facing Highest Suicide Rates" (press release), Lakota People's Law Project, May 2016, https://www.lakotalaw.org/news/2016-05-12/native-americans-facing-highest-suicide-rates.

20. Andres J. Azuero, Dan Arreaza-Kaufman, Jeanette Coriat, Stefano Tassinari, Annette Faria, Camilo Castañeda-Cardona, and Diego Rosselli, "Suicide in the Indigenous Population of Latin America: A Systemic Review," *Revista colombiana de psiquiatria* 46, no. 4 (2017), http://www.redalyc.org/pdf/806/80654035008.pdf.

21. Jonathan Watts, "Brazil Tribe Plagued by One of the Highest Suicide Rates in the World," *Guardian*, October 10, 2013, https://www.theguardian.com/world/2013/oct/10/suicide-rates-high-brazil-tribe.

22. Australian Bureau of Statistics (website), "3303.0 – Causes of Death, Australia, 2016," http://www.abs.gov.au/ausstats/abs@.nsf/mf/3303.0.

23. Ernest Hunter and Helen Milroy, "Aboriginal and Torres Strait Islander Suicide in Context," *Archives of Suicide Research* 10, no. 2 (2006), 141–57.

24. UN Permanent Forum on Indigenous Issues, 14th Session. "Concept Note for Discussion," 2015.

25. World Health Organization (website), "Health Impact Assessment: The Determinants of Health," http://www.who.int/hia/evidence/doh/en/.

26. Interview with Murray Sinclair, September 4, 2018.

27. Charles Mann, *1491: New Revelations of the Americas Before Columbus*, 2nd ed. (New York: Vintage Books, 2003), 15.

28. Neil Kent, *The Sámi Peoples of the North: A Social and Cultural History* (London: C. Hurst, 2014), 14.

29. American Museum of Natural History (website), "Social Darwinism," https://www.amnh.org/exhibitions/darwin/evolution-today/social-darwinism/.

30. Thomas King, *The Truth About Stories: A Native Narrative* (Toronto: House of Anansi Press, 2003), 106.

31. Bruce Pascoe, *Dark Emu: Aboriginal Australia and the Birth of Agriculture* (Melbourne: Scribe, 2018), 178.

32. Jim Dumont, *Indigenous Intelligence* (Sudbury: University of Sudbury, 2006), 1.

33. Ibid.

34. Laurentian University (website), "Our Tricultural Mandate," https://laurentian.ca/faculty/arts/our-tricultural-mandate.

35. Subsequent quotes and paraphrases from Dumont's lecture are from Dumont, *Indigenous Intelligence*, particularly 2, 4–6, 12, and 21.

36. Johan Turi, *Turi's Book of Lappland* (original title *Muittalus Samid Birra*), ed. and Danish trans. Emilie Demant Hatt; English trans. E. Gee Nash (London: Jonathan Cape, 1931), 11.

37. Kent, *The Sámi Peoples of the North*, 20; Noel D. Broadbent, *Lapps and Labyrinths: Saami Prehistory, Colonization and Cultural Resilience* (Washington, DC: Smithsonian Institution, 2010).

38. This and subsequent quotes from *Turi's Book of Lappland* are from 11–12, 19, 20, 24, 65, and 106–9.

39. Pascoe, *Dark Emu*, 104.

40. Ibid., 41.

41. Ibid., 104.

42. Ibid., 151.

43. Timothy R. Pauketat, *Cahokia: Ancient America's Great City on the Mississippi* (New York: Viking Penguin, 2009), 3.

44. Mann, *1491*, 288–89.

45. Ibid., 13.

46. Mississaugas of the New Credit First Nation (website), "Community Profile," http://mncfn.ca/about-mncfn/community-profile/.

47. Toronto's Historical Plaques (website), "The Ashbridge Estate," http://torontoplaques.com/Pages/Ashbridge_Estate.html.

48. Ojibwe (website), "Basic Ojibwe Words and Phrases," http://www.ojibwe.org/home/pdf/Ojibwe_Beginner_Dictionary.pdf.

CHAPTER 2: BIG BROTHER'S HUNGER

1. Tanya Talaga, "Rafting Down the Albany River to the Ring of Fire," *Toronto Star*, June 10, 2011, https://www.thestar.com/news/canada/2011/06/10/rafting_down_the_albany_river_to_the_ring_of_fire.html.

2. Jorge Barrera, "Ottawa Initially Fought St. Anne's Residential School Electric Chair Compensation Claims," CBC News, December 2, 2017, https://www.cbc.ca/news/indigenous/st-annes-residential-school-electric-chair-compensation-fight-1.4429594.

3. "Boreal Forests Called 'Northern Lungs of the World,'" CBC News, September 23, 2002, https://www.cbc.ca/news/technology/boreal-forests-called-northern-lungs-of-the-world-1.323586.

4. Tanya Talaga, "Cree Community Looks on Warily as De Beers Scours North for Diamonds," *Toronto Star*, October 10, 2015, https://www.thestar.com/news/insight/2015/10/10/cree-community-looks-on-warily-as-de-beers-eyes-new-diamond-mine.html.

5. Truth and Reconciliation Commission of Canada, *What We Have Learned: Principles of Truth and Reconciliation* (Winnipeg: Truth and Reconciliation Commission of Canada, 2015), 17–18,

http://www.trc.ca/websites/trcinstitution/File/2015/Findings/Principles%20of%20Truth%20and%20Reconciliation.pdf.

6. Kathryn Beck, "For as Long as the Rivers Flow," trans. Annie Ashamock (Nishnawbe Aski Nation, 2005), 2, 7, http://community.matawa.on.ca/wp-content/uploads/2013/12/For-as-Long-as-the-River-Flows-NAN-Treaty-9.pdf.

7. Gilder Lehrman Institute of American History (website), "History Now: The Doctrine of Discovery, 1493," https://www.gilderlehrman.org/content/doctrine-discovery-1493.

8. Truth and Reconciliation Commission, *What We Have Learned*, 18.

9. James Laxer, *Tecumseh and Brock: The War of 1812* (Toronto: House of Anansi Press, 2012), 23.

10. Timothy Egan, "The Nation: Mending a Trail of Broken Treaties," *New York Times*, June 25, 2000, https://www.nytimes.com/2000/06/25/weekinreview/the-nation-mending-a-trail-of-broken-treaties.html.

11. Laxer, *Tecumseh and Brock*, 23; J. Weston Phippen, "'Kill Every Buffalo You Can! Every Buffalo Dead Is an Indian Gone,'" *Atlantic*, May 13, 2016, https://www.theatlantic.com/national/archive/2016/05/the-buffalo-killers/482349/.

12. Geni (website), "Indian Wars: Red Stick War, 1813–1814," https://www.geni.com/projects/Indian-Wars-Red-Stick-War-1813-1814/1595; David Christopher, "Muscogee Creek History in Oklahoma," *Oklahoman*, June 29, 2010, https://newsok.com/article/3472197/muscogee-creek-history-in-oklahoma.

13. Laxer, *Tecumseh and Brock*, 226.

14. Michael D. Green, *The Politics of Indian Removal: Creek Government and Society in Crisis* (Lincoln: University of Nebraska Press, 1985), 43, cited in Laxer, *Tecumseh and Brock*, 226.

15. Cherokee Nation (website), "A Brief History of the Trail of Tears," http://www.cherokee.org/About-The-Nation/History/Trail-of-Tears/A-Brief-History-of-the-Trail-of-Tears; Library of Congress (website), "Primary Documents in American History: Indian

Removal Act," https://www.loc.gov/rr/program/bib/ourdocs/indian.html.

16. Truth and Reconciliation Commission, *What We Have Learned*, 17.

17. Phippen, "'Kill Every Buffalo.'"

18. Evan Andrews, "9 Things You May Not Know about William Tecumseh Sherman," History Channel (website), November 14, 2014, https://www.history.com/news/9-things-you-may-not-know-about-william-tecumseh-sherman.

19. Phippen, "'Kill Every Buffalo.'"

20. David M. Buerge, "Chief Seattle and Chief Joseph: From Indians to Icons," University of Washington Libraries Digital Collections, https://content.lib.washington.edu/aipnw/buerge2.html#joseph.

21. Biography (website), "Chief Joseph," https://www.biography.com/people/chief-joseph-9358227.

22. PBS (website), "New Perspectives on the West: Chief Joseph," https://www.pbs.org/weta/thewest/people/a_c/chiefjoseph.htm.

23. "Chief Joseph Dead: 'The Napoleon of Indians,' Whom Gen. Miles Finally Subdued," *New York Times*, September 24, 1904.

24. Howard B. Leavitt, ed., *First Encounters: Native Voices on the Coming of the Europeans* (Santa Barbara, CA: Greenwood, 2010), 133.

25. Ibid., 138.

26. "Chief Joseph Dead," *New York Times*.

27. Global Policy Forum (website), "US Territorial Acquisition," https://www.globalpolicy.org/component/content/article/155-history/25993.html.

28. Michael R. Haines and Richard H. Steckel, *A Population History of North America* (Cambridge: Cambridge University Press, 2000), 24.

29. Charla Bear, "American Indian Boarding Schools Haunt Many," NPR, May 12, 2008, https://www.npr.org/templates/story/story.php?storyId=16516865.

30. Ibid.

31. First Nations Child and Family Caring Society of Canada, "The Legacy of Duncan Campbell Scott: More Than Just a Canadian Poet," July 2016, https://fncaringsociety.com/sites/default/files/Duncan%20Campbell%20Scott%20Information%20Sheet_FINAL.pdf.

32. Indigenous and Northern Affairs Canada (website), "Treaty Texts: Treaty No. 9," https://www.aadnc-aandc.gc.ca/eng/1100100028863/1100100028864.

33. Ibid.

34. John S. Long, *Treaty No. 9: Making the Agreement to Share the Land in Far Northern Ontario in 1905* (Montreal: McGill-Queen's University Press, 2010), 19, 20, 23.

35. James Morrison, "Treaty Research Report, Treaty No. 9 (1905–1906)," Treaties and Historical Research Centre, Indian and Northern Affairs Canada, 1986, https://www.aadnc-aandc.gc.ca/eng/1100100028859/1100100028861; Long, *Treaty No. 9*, 44.

36. Long, *Treaty No. 9*, 44.

37. Indigenous and Northern Affairs, "Treaty No. 9."

38. Diary of Treaty 9 Commissioner D. G. W. MacMartin, 1905, MacMartin Papers, Miscellaneous Collection, Locator 2325.9, Queen's University Archives, transcribed by Ian Martyn and Associates, 2009, 12.

39. Truth and Reconciliation Commission, *What We Have Learned*, 25.

40. Xavier Kataquapit, "MacMartin's Diary Sheds New Light on Treaty #9," *Nation News*, February 25, 2011, http://www.nationnews.ca/macmartins-diary-sheds-new-light-on-treaty-9/.

41. Lenny Carpenter, "Mushkegowuk Launches Lawsuit on Treaty Promises," *Wawatay News*, August 8, 2013, http://www.wawatay news.ca/home/mushkegowuk-launches-lawsuit-treaty-promises.

42. Long, *Treaty No. 9*, 38.

43. Truth and Reconciliation Commission, *What We Have Learned*, 7, 15.

44. First Nations Caring Society, "Legacy of Duncan Campbell Scott."

45. Truth and Reconciliation Commission, *What We Have Learned*, 6.

46. Chinta Puxley, "How Many First Nations Kids Died in Residential Schools? Justice Murray Sinclair Says Canada Needs Answers," *Toronto Star*, May 31, 2015, https://www.thestar.com/news/canada/2015/05/31/how-many-first-nations-kids-died-in-residential-schools-justice-murray-sinclair-says-canada-needs-answers.html.

47. Inuit Tapiriit Kanatami (website), "Who We Are," https://www.itk.ca/national-voice-for-communities-in-the-canadian-arctic/.

48. Travel Nunavut (website), "Weather & Climate," https://www.nunavuttourism.com/plan-and-book/visitor-information/weather-climate/.

49. Unikkaarvik Visitor Centre, Iqaluit, Nunavut.

50. Travel Nunavut, "Weather and Climate."

51. Sue Hamilton, "Defining the Inuit Dog: History," The Fan Hitch (website), http://thefanhitch.org/theISD/History.html.

52. Arthur J. Ray, *I Have Lived Here Since the World Began: An Illustrated History of Canada's Native People*, rev. ed. (Toronto: Key Porter Books, 2005), 268–75.

53. Adam Shoalts, "Reverse Colonialism: How the Inuit Conquered the Vikings," *Canadian Geographic*, March 8, 2011, https://www.canadiangeographic.ca/article/reverse-colonialism-how-inuit-conquered-vikings.

54. Unikkaarvik Visitor Centre.

55. Dave Dean, "The RCMP and Quebec's Provincial Police Nearly Killed Off the Inuit Sled Dog," *Vice*, September 25, 2013, https://www.vice.com/en_ca/article/zn8wy8/the-rcmp-and-quebecs-provincial-police-nearly-killed-off-the-inuit-sled-dog.

56. Qikiqtani Truth Commission, "Analysis of the RCMP Sled Dog Report: Thematic Reports and Special Studies, 1950–1975," (Iqaluit: Inhabit Media, 2013),10, https://www.qtcommission.ca/

sites/default/files/public/thematic_reports/thematic_reports_english_rcmp_sled_dog.pdf.

57. Ibid., 11–12, 15.

58. Ibid., 15, 18, 20.

59. Natan Obed, speech at Upstream conference, Ottawa, March 4, 2018.

60. Marshall C. Eakin, *The History of Latin America: Collision of Cultures* (New York: St. Martin's Griffin, 2007), 88.

61. Ibid.

62. Norman Lewis, "Genocide," *Sunday Times Magazine*, February 23, 1969, 43, http://assets.survivalinternational.org/documents/1094/genocide-norman-lewis-1969.pdf.

63. Eakin, *Collision of Cultures*, 89.

64. Ibid.

65. Ibid., 91.

66. Lewis, "Genocide," 43.

67. Ibid., 42, 43.

68. Ibid., 42.

69. Survival International (website), "The Guarani," https://www.survivalinternational.org/tribes/guarani.

70. Ibid.

71. Survival International, "Violations of the Rights of the Guarani of Mato Grosso do Sul State: A Survival International Report to the UN Committee on the Elimination of Racial Discrimination," March 2010, 6, http://assets.survivalinternational.org/documents/207/Guarani_report_English_MARCH.pdf.

72. Chris Lang, "Open Letter from Amnesty International to Brazil's President about Violations of the Rights of the Guarani-Kaiowá Indigenous People," REDD-Monitor, November 6, 2015, http://www.redd-monitor.org/2015/11/06/open-letter-from-amnesty-international-to-brazils-president-about-violations-of-the-rights-of-the-guarani-kaiowa-indigenous-people/.

73. Survival International, "Violations of the Rights of the Guarani," 5.

74. Ibid., 4.

75. International Federation for Human Rights (FIDH), "Brazil: Killing of Mr. Semião Fernandes Vilhalva, One of the Leaders of the Guarani-Kaiowá Indigenous People in Brazil," September 10, 2015, https://www.fidh.org/en/region/americas/brazil/brazil-killing-of-mr-semiao-fernandes-vilhalva-one-of-the-leaders-of#.

76. Survival International, "Brazil: Guarani Man Assassinated by Gunmen as Tensions Rise," September 2, 2015, https://www.survivalinternational.org/news/10891.

77. Lang, "Open Letter."

78. Wyre Davies, "Brazil's Guarani-Kaiowa Tribe Allege Genocide over Land Disputes," BBC News, September 8, 2015, https://www.bbc.com/news/world-latin-america-34183280.

79. Survival International, "Violations of the Rights of the Guarani," 7.

80. Ibid., 4.

81. Ibid., 7.

82. *Indigenous Peoples Atlas of Canada* (website), "Métis: Communities," https://indigenouspeoplesatlasofcanada.ca/article/communities/; Chelsea Vowel, *Indigenous Writes: A Guide to First Nations, Métis & Inuit Issues in Canada* (Winnipeg: HighWater Press / Portage & Main Press, 2016), 39.

83. Survival International, "Violations of the Rights of the Guarani," 1–2.

84. Lang, "Open Letter."

85. Vanessa Barbara, "The Genocide of Brazil's Indians," *New York Times*, May 29, 2017, https://www.nytimes.com/2017/05/29/opinion/the-genocide-of-brazils-indians.html.

86. Andreia Verdélio, "Some 11 Thousand Brazilians Commit Suicide Every Year," Agência Brasil, September 23, 2017, http://agenciabrasil.ebc.com.br/en/geral/noticia/2017-09/some-11-thousand-brazilians-commit-suicide-every-year.

87. Christina Lamb, "Rising Suicides Cut a Swath Through Amazon's Children," *Telegraph*, November 19, 2000, https://www.telegraph.co.uk/news/worldnews/asia/1374881/Rising-suicides-cut-a-swath-through-Amazons-children.html.

88. Larry Rohter, "Diamonds' Glitter Fades for a Brazilian Tribe," *New York Times*, December 29, 2006.

89. Five Books (website), "The Best Books on Brazil: Recommended by Larry Rohter," https://fivebooks.com/best-books/brazil-larry-rohter/.

90. Shasta Darlington, "'Uncontacted' Amazon Tribe Members Reported Killed in Brazil," *New York Times*, September 10, 2017, https://www.nytimes.com/2017/09/10/world/americas/brazil-amazon-tribe-killings.html.

91. Dom Phillips, "Footage of Sole Survivor of Amazon Tribe Emerges," *Guardian*, July 19, 2018, https://www.theguardian.com/world/2018/jul/19/footage-sole-survivor-amazon-tribe-emerges-brazil.

CHAPTER 3: THE THIRD SPACE

1. Seven Generations Education Institute (website), "Mino Bimaadizwin: Principles for Anishinaabe Education," http://www.7generations.org/wp-content/uploads/2015/03/AMB-Booklet-3.pdf.

2. Royal Commission into Institutional Responses to Child Sexual Abuse, "A Brief Guide to the Final Report: Aboriginal and Torres Strait Islander Communities," 2017, 2, https://www.childabuseroyalcommission.gov.au/sites/default/files/a_brief_guide_to_the_final_report.pdf.

3. "Australia Child Abuse Inquiry Finds 'Serious Failings,'" BBC News, December 15, 2017, https://www.bbc.com/news/world-australia-42361874.

4. Nick McKenzie, Richard Baker, and Jane Lee, "Church's Suicide Victims," *Age*, April 13, 2012, https://www.theage.com.au/

national/victoria/churchs-suicide-victims-20120412-1wwox. html.

5. "Australia Child Abuse Inquiry," BBC News.

6. Royal Commission into Institutional Responses to Child Sexual Abuse, *Final Report: Recommendations* (Barton, ACT: Commonwealth of Australia, 2017), https://www. childabuseroyalcommission.gov.au/sites/default/files/final_ report_-_recommendations.pdf; "Child Sexual Abuse Royal Commission: Recommendations and Statistics at a Glance," *Guardian*, December 15, 2017, https://www.theguardian. com/australia-news/2017/dec/15/child-sexual-abuse-royal-commission-recommendations-and-statistics-at-a-glance.

7. Royal Commission into Institutional Responses, "Brief Guide," 2, 4.

8. Ian Lloyd Neubauer, "Australian Child Protection Accused of Repeating Sins of 'Stolen Generations,'" *Time*, March 11, 2014, http://time.com/19431/australian-child-protection-accused-of-repeating-sins-of-stolen-generations/.

9. Karina Marlow, "Explainer: The Stolen Generations," National Indigenous Television, December 1, 2016, https://www.sbs.com. au/nitv/explainer/explainer-stolen-generations; Human Rights and Equal Opportunity Commission (Australia), *Bringing Them Home: Report of the National Inquiry into the Separation of Aboriginal and Torres Strait Islander Children from Their Families* (Sydney: Commonwealth of Australia, 1997), https://www.humanrights. gov.au/sites/default/files/content/pdf/social_justice/bringing_ them_home_report.pdf; Australian Institute of Aboriginal and Torres Strait Islander Studies (website), "Remembering the Mission Days: Stories from the Aborigines' Inland Missions," https://aiatsis.gov.au/exhibitions/remembering-mission-days.

10. Human Rights and Equal Opportunity Commission, *Bringing Them Home*, 4.

11. Marlow, "Explainer."

12. Calla Wahlquist, "Australia's Stolen Generations: A Legacy of Intergenerational Pain and Broken Bonds," *Guardian*, May 24, 2017,

https://www.theguardian.com/australia-news/2017/may/25/australias-stolen-generations-a-legacy-of-intergenerational-pain-and-broken-bonds.

13. "Australia Is Failing to Improve Indigenous Lives, Report Shows," BBC News, February 14, 2017, https://www.bbc.com/news/world-australia-38965545.

14. "Australia Accused of 'Effectively Abandoning' Indigenous Goals," BBC News, February 8, 2018, https://www.bbc.com/news/world-australia-42983877.

15. Mushkegowuk Council, *The People's Inquiry into Our Suicide Pandemic*, written and submitted October 27, 2014, published 2016, http://caid.ca/MusCouInq2016_Rep.pdf.

16. Wapekeka First Nation (website), www.wapekeka.ca.

17. "Fire Destroys the Reverend Eleazer Memorial School in Wapekeka FN," *Net News Ledger*, May 14, 2015, http://www.netnewsledger.com/2015/05/14/fire-destroys-the-reverend-eleazar-winter-memorial-school-in-wapekeka-fn/; Nishnawbe Aski Nation (website), "2016 Photo Gallery: 2016 Wapekeka School," February 3, 2016, http://www.nan.on.ca/article/2016-wapekeka-school-grand-opening-2214.asp.

18. *R v Ralph Rowe*, 2012, ONCJ, Proceedings before the Honourable Justice D. Fraser, August 9, 2012, Kenora, Ontario.

19. Jody Porter, "Class Action Suit Launched Against Pedophile Ex-priest Ralph Rowe," CBC News, May 11, 2017, https://www.cbc.ca/news/canada/thunder-bay/ralph-rowe-lawsuit-1.4111104.

20. Interview with Stephanie Harrington, June 3, 2018.

21. "Ralph Rowe on Trial on New Charges" (press release), Nishnawbe Aski Nation, April 15, 2009, http://www.nan.on.ca/upload/documents/com-2009-04-15-ralph-rowe-trial.pdf.

22. *R v Ralph Rowe*.

23. Interview with Anna Betty Achneepineskum, April 16, 2018.

24. Kristy Kirkup, Canadian Press, "Confront Scourge of Sexual Abuse, Stand Up for Children, Inuit Leaders Demand," CBC News,

November 9, 2016, https://www.cbc.ca/news/canada/north/inuit-leaders-child-sexual-abuse-1.3843250.

25. Federation of Sovereign Indigenous Nations, *Saskatchewan First Nations Suicide Prevention Strategy* (Saskatoon, SK: FSIN, 2018), 8–9, https://www.fsin.com/wp-content/uploads/2018/05/SFNSPS-FINAL-2018-May-24.pdf.

26. Ibid., 12.

27. Interview with Maggie Pettis, May 1, 2018.

28. Gerry Georgatos, "77 Aboriginal Suicides in South Australia Alone," *Stringer,* October 4, 2013, http://thestringer.com.au/77-aboriginal-suicides-in-south-australia-alone-4994#.W3GueZNKjMU.

29. Inuit Tapiriit Kanatami, *National Inuit Suicide Prevention Strategy* (Ottawa: ITK, 2016), 4, https://www.itk.ca/wp-content/uploads/2016/07/ITK-National-Inuit-Suicide-Prevention-Strategy-2016.pdf.

30. Inuit Tapiriit Kanatami, "Protective Factors," https://www.itk.ca/preventing-suicide-among-inuit/protective-factors/.

31. Inuit Tapiriit Kanatami, *Prevention Strategy*, 6.

32. Eliza Racine, "Native Americans Facing Highest Suicide Rates" (press release), Lakota People's Law Project, May 2016, https://www.lakotalaw.org/news/2016-05-12/native-americans-facing-highest-suicide-rates.

33. UNICEF, *Report on the Situation of Children and Adolescents in Brazil* (Brasilia: unicef Brazil, 2003), 23, https://www.unicef.org/brazil/english/siab_english.pdf.

34. Vanessa Barbara, "The Genocide of Brazil's Indians," *New York Times,* May 29, 2017, https://www.nytimes.com/2017/05/29/opinion/the-genocide-of-brazils-indians.html.

35. Interview with Janete Morais, August 3, 2018.

36. June C. Strickland, "Suicide among American Indian, Alaskan Native, and Canadian Aboriginal Youth: Advancing the Research Agenda," *International Journal of Mental Health* 25, no. 4 (1996–97): 13.

37. Ibid.

38. Ben Spurr, "How the Attawapiskat Suicide Unfolded," *Toronto Star*, April 18, 2016, https://www.thestar.com/news/canada/2016/04/18/how-the-attawapiskat-suicide-crisis-unfolded.html.

39. A. Silviken, T. Haldorsen, and S. Kvernmo, "Suicide among Indigenous Sami in Arctic Norway, 1970–1998," *European Journal of Epidemiology* 21, no. 9 (2006): 708; Strickland, "Suicide," 13; C. McHugh, A. Campbell, M. Chapman, and S. Balaratnasingam, "Increasing Indigenous Self-Harm and Suicide in the Kimberley: An Audit of the 2005–2014 Data," *Medical Journal of Australia* 205, no. 1 (July 2016): 33, https://www.mja.com.au/system/files/issues/205_01/10.5694mja15.01368.pdf.

40. R. J. McQuaid, A. Bombay, O. A. McInnis, C. Humeny, K. Matheson, and H. Anisman, "Suicide Ideation and Attempts among First Nations Peoples Living On-Reserve in Canada: The Intergenerational and Cumulative Effects of Indian Residential Schools," *Canadian Journal of Psychiatry* 62, no. 6 (2017): 422–30.

41. Michael J. Chandler and Christopher E. Lalonde, "Cultural Continuity as a Protective Factor against Suicide in First Nations Youth," *Horizons* 10, no. 1 (2008): 68–72, https://www.researchgate.net/publication/239921354.

42. Michael J. Chandler and Christopher E. Lalonde, "Cultural Continuity as a Hedge against Suicide in Canada's First Nations," *Transcultural Psychiatry* 35, no. 2 (June 1998): 191, quoted in Jack Hicks, "A Critical Analysis of Myth-Perpetuating Research on Suicide Prevention," *Northern Public Affairs* 5, no. 3 (April 2018): 44.

43. Hicks, "Critical Analysis," 44.

44. Chandler and Lalonde, "Cultural Continuity as a Protective Factor."

45. Ibid.

46. Anne Russell, "Back to the Land: Building Resiliency by Connecting Aboriginal Youth to Place," UFV Today (website), July 11, 2016, https://blogs.ufv.ca/blog/2016/07/back-to-the-land-building-resiliency-by-connecting-aboriginal-youth-to-place/.

47. "Youth Suicide Pact Triggers Call for Action in Vancouver," CBC News, November 23, 2012, https://www.cbc.ca/news/canada/

british-columbia/youth-suicide-pact-triggers-call-for-action-in-vancouver-1.1165251.

48. Patrick Johnston, "Revisiting the 'Sixties Scoop' of Indigenous Children," *Policy Options*, July 26, 2016, http://policyoptions.irpp.org/magazines/july-2016/revisiting-the-sixties-scoop-of-indigenous-children/.

49. Indigenous Foundations, University of British Columbia (website), "Sixties Scoop," https://indigenousfoundations.arts.ubc.ca/sixties_scoop/.

50. Ibid.

51. Johnston, "Revisiting the 'Sixties Scoop.'"

52. John Paul Tasker, "Jane Philpott Unveils 6-Point Plan to Improve 'Perverse' First Nations Child Welfare System," CBC News, January 25, 2018, https://www.cbc.ca/news/politics/jane-philpott-six-point-plan-first-nations-child-welfare-1.4503264.

53. Interview with Spensy Pimentel, August 7, 2018.

54. Henry Minde, "Assimilation of the Sami: Implementation and Consequences," paper 196, Aboriginal Policy Research Consortium International (APRCi), 2005, 7–9, https://ir.lib.uwo.ca/cgi/viewcontent.cgi?referer=https://www.google.com/&httpsredir=1&article=1248&context=aprci.

55. Ibid., 8–10.

56. Arctic Centre, University of Lapland, "Stereotypes Die Hard!," September 22, 2015, https://arcticanthropology.org/2015/09/22/stereotypes-die-hard/.

57. Minde, "Assimilation of the Sami," 21.

58. Robert Paine, *Herds of the Tundra: A Portrait of Reindeer Pastoralism* (Washington, DC: Smithsonian Institution Press, 1994), 11, cited in Scott Forrest, "Territoriality in State–Sámi Relations," 1996, http://arcticcircle.uconn.edu/HistoryCulture/Sami/samisf.html; Joan Sullivan, "Anthropologist's Research Ranged from Newfoundland Speech to West Bank Jews," *Globe and Mail*, July 17, 2010, http://v1.theglobeandmail.com/servlet/story/LAC.20100717.OBPAINEATL/BDAStory/BDA/deaths.

59. The account that follows, including direct quotes, is from an interview with Simon Issát Marainen, May 31, 2018.

CHAPTER 4: "I BREATHE FOR THEM"

1. Scott-McKay-Bain Health Panel, *From Here to There: Steps along the Way* (Sioux Lookout, ON, 1989), 10, http://www.slmhc.on.ca/assets/files/From_Here_to_There_-_Steps_Along_the_Way.pdf.

2. Noni E. MacDonald, Richard Stanwick, and Andrew Lynk, "Canada's Shameful History of Nutrition Research on Residential School Children: The Need for Strong Medical Ethics in Aboriginal Health Research," *Paediatrics & Child Health* 19, no. 2 (2014): 64, https://www.ncbi.nlm.nih.gov/pmc/articles/PMC3941673/.

3. Interview with Ian Mosby, *As It Happens*, CBC Radio, July 16, 2013, https://www.cbc.ca/radio/asithappens/wednesday-aboriginal-experiments-zetas-cartel-leader-obit-don-smith-1.2941800/food-historian-discovers-federal-government-experimented-on-aboriginal-children-during-and-after-wwii-1.2941801.

4. Richard Chenhall and Kate Senior, "Those Young People All Crankybella: Indigenous Youth Mental Health and Globalization," *International Journal of Mental Health* 38, no. 3 (2009): 28–43.

5. Royal Commission into Institutional Responses to Child Sexual Abuse, *Final Report: Preface and Executive Summary* (Barton, ACT: Commonwealth of Australia, 2017), 13, https://www.childabuseroyalcommission.gov.au/sites/default/files/final_report_-_preface_and_executive_summary.pdf.

6. Melissa Sweet, Kerry McCallum, Lynore Geia, and Kathleen Musulin, "Acknowledge the Brutal History of Indigenous Health Care — for Healing," *Conversation*, September 21, 2016, https://theconversation.com/acknowledge-the-brutal-history-of-indigenous-health-care-for-healing-64295.

7. Social Health Reference Group for National Aboriginal and Torres Strait Islander Health Council and National Mental Health Working Group, *Social and Emotional Well Being Framework: A National Strategic Framework for Aboriginal and Torres Strait*

Islander Peoples' Mental Health and Social and Emotional Well Being, 2004–2009 (Surry Hills, NSW: Aboriginal Health and Medical Research Council of New South Wales, 2004), https://www.ahmrc.org.au/media/resources/social-emotional-wellbeing/mental-health/328-national-strategic-framework-for-aboriginal-and-torres-strait-islander-peoples-mental-health-and-social-and-emotional-well-being-2004-2009/file.html.

8. Australia, "Aboriginal Peoples and Torres Strait Islanders," in *Pathways of Recovery: Preventing Further Episodes of Mental Illness* (Department of Health, Commonwealth of Australia, 2006), http://health.gov.au/internet/publications/publishing.nsf/Content/mental-pubs-p-mono-toc~mental-pubs-p-mono-pop~mental-pubs-p-mono-pop-atsi.

9. Office of the Surgeon General, Center for Mental Health Services, and National Institute of Mental Health, *Mental Health: Culture, Race, and Ethnicity; A Supplement to Mental Health: A Report of the Surgeon General* (Rockville, MD: Substance Abuse and Mental Health Services Administration, 2001), https://www.ncbi.nlm.nih.gov/books/NBK44243/; American Psychiatric Association, "Mental Health Disparities: American Indians and Alaska Natives" (fact sheet), 2017, https://www.psychiatry.org/File%20Library/Psychiatrists/Cultural-Competency/Mental-Health-Disparities/Mental-Health-Facts-for-American-Indian-Alaska-Natives.pdf.

10. Indian Health Service, "Fact Sheet: Disparities," April 2017, https://www.ihs.gov/newsroom/factsheets/disparities/.

11. Margo Lianne Greenwood and Sarah Naomi de Leeuw, "Social Determinants of Health and the Future Well-Being of Aboriginal Children in Canada," *Paediatrics & Child Health* 17, no. 7 (2012): 381–84, https://www.ncbi.nlm.nih.gov/pmc/articles/PMC3448539/.

12. Travis Heath, "7 Interesting Facts about Sioux Lookout," *Northern Ontario Travel*, August 22, 2015, https://www.northernontario.travel/sunset-country/7-interesting-facts-about-sioux-lookout.

13. Municipality of Sioux Lookout (website), "Legend of Sioux Lookout," http://www.siouxlookout.ca/en/discover-the-hub/legend-of-sioux-lookout.asp; Sioux Lookout Chamber of

Commerce (website), "The Legend of Sioux Lookout," adapted from an article by Nan Shipley, https://www.siouxlookout.com/about-sioux-lookout.

14. Maureen K. Lux, *Separate Beds: A History of Indian Hospitals in Canada, 1920s–1980s* (Toronto: University of Toronto Press, 2016), 31–32.

15. Maureen K. Lux, "Indian Hospitals in Canada," in *The Canadian Encylopedia Online*, July 17, 2017, https://www.thecanadian encyclopedia.ca/en/article/indian-hospitals-in-canada/.

16. Canadian Public Health Association (website), "TB and Aboriginal People," https://www.cpha.ca/tb-and-aboriginal-people.

17. First Nations Child and Family Caring Society of Canada, "Dr. Peter Henderson Bryce: A Story of Courage," July 2016, https://fncaringsociety.com/sites/default/files/Dr.%20Peter%20 Henderson%20Bryce%20Information%20Sheet.pdf.

18. Ibid.

19. South African History Online (website), "A History of Apartheid in South Africa," https://www.sahistory.org.za/article/history-apartheid-south-africa.

20. History Channel (website), "Apartheid," October 7, 2010, https://www.history.com/topics/apartheid.

21. *Encyclopaedia Britannica Online*, s.v. "Apartheid," https://www.britannica.com/topic/apartheid.

22. Gloria Galloway, "Chiefs Reflect on Apartheid and First Nations as Atleo Visits Mandela Memorial," *Globe and Mail*, December 11, 2013, https://www.theglobeandmail.com/news/politics/chiefs-reflect-on-apartheid-and-first-nations-as-atleo-visits-mandela-memorial/article15902124/.

23. Lux, "Indian Hospitals."

24. Lux, *Separate Beds*, 31–32.

25. Indigenous Corporate Training (website), "A Brief Look at Indian Hospitals in Canada," June 3, 2017, https://www.ictinc.ca/blog/a-brief-look-at-indian-hospitals-in-canada-0.

26. Lux, "Indian Hospitals."

27. Lux, *Separate Beds*, 75.

28. Ibid., 96.

29. Ibid., 80–81.

30. Ibid.

31. Ibid., 99–101.

32. Lux, "Indian Hospitals."

33. Ibid.

34. Indigenous Corporate Training, "Brief Look at Indian Hospitals."

35. Canadian Public Health Association, "TB and Aboriginal People."

36. Scott-McKay-Bain Health Panel, *From Here to There*, 9.

37. "Hospital offers holistic healing," *Wawatay News*, October 28, 2010.

38. Scott-McKay-Bain Health Panel, *From Here to There*, 9.

39. Ibid., 14.

40. Meno Ya Win Health Centre (website), "Sioux Lookout Four Party Hospital Services Agreement," http://www.slmhc.on.ca/hospital-services-agreement.

41. Nishnawbe Aski Nation (website), "Backgrounder: Health and Public Health Emergency," http://www.nan.on.ca/upload/documents/comms-2016-02-24-backgrounder-health-eme.pdf.

42. This and subsequent quotes from Alexander Caudarella are from an interview and email correspondence with Caudarella, April 8 and September 8, 2018, respectively.

43. United Nations General Assembly, "Declaration on the Rights of Indigenous Peoples" (Geneva: United Nations, March 2008), 9, https://www.un.org/esa/socdev/unpfii/documents/DRIPS_en.pdf.

44. "Underlying Issues," chapter 5 in *Bringing Them Home: Report of the National Inquiry into the Separation of Aboriginal and Torres Strait Islander Children from Their Families* (Sydney: Human Rights and Equal Opportunity Commission, 1997), https://www.humanrights.gov.au/publications/bringing-them-home-chapter-25.

45. "Brazil: Homicides of Children and Teenagers Double in 20 Years: unicef Report," (press release), unicef, July 16, 2015, https://www.unicef.org/media/media_82554.html.

46. Sabine Dolan, "Reaching Out to Brazil's Most Disadvantaged: The Plight of Indigenous Children," (press release), unicef, April 8, 2005, https://www.unicef.org/infobycountry/brazil_25958.html.

47. Assembly of First Nations, "Closing the Gap: 2015 Federal Election Priorities for First Nations and Canada" (Ottawa: AFM, September 2, 2015), 8, http://www.afn.ca/uploads/files/closing-the-gap.pdf.

48. Ibid.

49. Isabella Kwai and Tacey Rychter, "'I Can't Breathe': Video of Indigenous Australian's Prison Death Stirs Outrage," *New York Times*, July 16, 2018, https://www.nytimes.com/2018/07/16/world/australia/i-cant-breathe-indigenous-australian-prison-death.html.

50. Ibid.

51. Jim Rankin, "Inmate in Solitary for Four Years Alarms Rights Commission," *Toronto Star*, October 19, 2016, https://www.thestar.com/news/canada/2016/10/19/inmate-in-solitary-for-four-years-alarms-rights-commission.html; Adrian Morrow and Patrick White, "Ontario Minister Refuses to Release Man from Solitary Who's Spent Four Years in Isolation," *Globe and Mail*, October 25, 2016, https://www.theglobeandmail.com/news/national/solitary-confinement-ontario-prisons-adam-capay/article32527317/.

52. Jody Porter, "No Mental Health Support Available for First Nations Artist Who Died in Jail, Chief Says," CBC News, February 15, 2017, https://www.cbc.ca/news/canada/thunder-bay/moses-beaver-dies-1.3983986.

53. Assembly of First Nations, "Closing the Gap," 8.

54. Josée Lavoie, "Policy Silences: Why Canada Needs a National First Nations, Inuit and Métis Health Policy," *International Journal of Circumpolar Health* 72, no. 10 (2013): https://www.ncbi.nlm.nih.gov/pmc/articles/PMC3875351/.

55. Government of Canada (website), "Canada Health Act," https://www.canada.ca/en/health-canada/services/health-care-system/canada-health-care-system-medicare/canada-health-act.html.

56. Canadian Press, "Ottawa to Pay for Travel Companion for Indigenous Women Giving Birth Away from Reserve," CBC News, April 9, 2017, https://www.cbc.ca/news/politics/indigenous-women-pregnancy-reserve-escort-policy-change-1.4063082.

57. "Brian Sinclair's Death 'Preventable' but Not Homicide, Says Inquest Report," CBC News, December 12, 2014, http://www.cbc.ca/news/canada/manitoba/brian-sinclair-s-death-preventable-but-not-homicide-says-inquest-report-1.2871025.

58. "Complete List: 63 Recommendations in the Brian Sinclair Inquest Report," *Winnipeg Free Press*, December 12, 2014, https://www.winnipegfreepress.com/local/Complete-list-63--285628851.html.

59. Office of the Auditor General of Canada, *Report 4: Access to Health Services for Remote First Nations Communities* (Ottawa: 2015 Spring Reports of the Auditor General of Canada), 4.9, http://www.oag-bvg.gc.ca/internet/English/parl_oag_201504_04_e_40350.html#hd3c.

60. Ibid., 4.66.

61. Ibid.

62. Michael Ferguson, "Opening Statement to the Standing Committee on Public Accounts," (Ottawa: 2015 Spring Reports of the Auditor General of Canada), http://www.oag-bvg.gc.ca/internet/English/osh_20150429_e_40484.html.

63. Auditor General, *Access to Health Services*, 4.90.

64. Janet Gordon, Mike Kirlew, Yoko Schreiber, Raphael Saginur, Natalie Bocking, Brittany Blakelock, Michelle Haavaldsrud, Christine Kennedy, Terri Farrell, Lloyd Douglas, and Len Kelly, "Acute Rheumatic Fever in First Nations Communities in Northwestern Ontario," *Canadian Family Physician* 61, no. 10 (2015): 881–86, http://www.cfp.ca/content/61/10/881.

65. Ontario Public Health Convention, 2019 program, "Session 44: Epidemic of Opioid Abuse in Remote First Nations in Northwest

Ontario," http://www.tophc.ca/session-44-epidemic-of-opioid-abuse-in-remote-first-nations-in-northwestern-ontario/.

66. Interview with Mike Kirlew, January 3, 2018.

67. This and subsequent quotes from Peter Voros are from an interview and email correspondence with Voros, April 2018 and September 5, 2018, respectively.

68. Federation of Sovereign Indigenous Nations, *Saskatchewan First Nations Suicide Prevention Strategy* (Saskatoon, SK: FSIN, 2018), 14, https://www.fsin.com/wp-content/uploads/2018/05/SFNSPS-FINAL-2018-May-24.pdf.

69. Ibid.

70. Ibid., 15.

71. Ibid., 17.

72. Allison Crawford and Jack Hicks, "Early Childhood Adversity as a Key Mechanism by Which Colonialism Is Mediated into Suicidal Behaviour," *Journal of Northern Public Affairs* 65, no. 3 (April 2018): 18–22.

73. Ibid.

74. Ibid.

75. Ibid.

76. Ibid., 20.

77. Sámi Norwegian National Advisory Unit on Mental Health and Substance Abuse and Saami Council, *Plan for Suicide Prevention among the Sámi People in Norway, Sweden and Finland* (Karasjok: SANKS, 2017), https://finnmarkssykehuset.no/documents/sanks/plan%20for%20suicide%20prevention%20among%20the%20sámi%20people%20in%20norway.pdf.

78. Anthony Ham and Oliver Berry, *Lonely Planet Norway*, 7th ed. (Footscray, VIC: Lonely Planet, 2018), 313.

79. Heather Carrie, Tim K. Mackey, and Sloane N. Laird, "Integrating Traditional Indigenous Medicine and Western Biomedicine into Health systems: A Review of Nicaraguan Health Policies and Miskitu Health Services," *International Journal of Equity Health*

14, no. 129 (2015), https://www.ncbi.nlm.nih.gov/pmc/articles/PMC4663733/.

80. "President Obama Announces U.S. Support for United Nations Declaration on the Rights of Indigenous Peoples," (press release), National Congress of American Indians, December 16, 2010, http://www.ncai.org/news/articles/2010/12/16/president-obama-announces-u-s-support-for-united-nations-declaration-on-the-rights-of-indigenous-peoples.

81. Gloria Galloway, "Canada Drops Opposition to UN Indigenous Rights Declaration," *Globe and Mail*, May 9, 2016, https://www.theglobeandmail.com/news/politics/canada-drops-objector-status-on-un-indigenous-rights-declaration/article29946223/.

82. Nahka Bertrand, "Romeo Saganash Speaks about undrip's Human Rights Application in Canadian Law," *Nation*, March 31, 2018, http://www.nationnews.ca/romeo-saganash-speaks-undrips-human-rights-application-canadian-law/.

CHAPTER 5: WE ARE NOT GOING ANYWHERE

1. Steve Heinrichs, *The Truth and Reconciliation Commission and Mennonite Church Canada* (Winnipeg: Mennonite Church Canada, 2012), 6, https://www.commonword.ca/FileDownload/19042/2012_MCCan_TRC_handout.pdf?t=1.

2. Donald J. Auger, *Indian Residential Schools in Ontario* (Nishnawbe Aski Nation, 2005), 193.

3. This and subsequent quotes are from an interview with Rance Christianson, September 7, 2018.

4. Julian N. Falconer, Molly Churchill, and Amanda Byrd, "Bureaucratic Immunity as a Barrier to Change: Dismantling the Structures at the Heart of the Indian Act." Paper presented at the determiNATION Summit, Ottawa, May 23, 2018, http://www.falconers.ca/wp-content/uploads/2018/05/determiNATION.Paper_.BureaucraticImmunity.Final_.22May2018.pdf.

5. Indigenous Foundations, University of British Columbia (website), "Constitution Act, 1982 Section 5," https://indigenousfoundations.arts.ubc.ca/constitution_act_1982_section_35/.

6. Interview with Jody Wilson-Raybould, *The House*, CBC Radio, February 17, 2018, https://www.cbc.ca/listen/shows/the-house/episode/15521280.

7. Minister Carolyn Bennett, speech during the Assembly of First Nations Special Chiefs, December 6, 2017, https://www.canada.ca/en/indigenous-northern-affairs/news/2017/12/speech_of_ministercarolynbennettduringtheassemblyoffirstnationss.html.

8. Mushkegowuk Council, *The People's Inquiry into Our Suicide Pandemic*, written and submitted October 27, 2014, published 2016, http://caid.ca/MusCouInq2016_Rep.pdf.

9. Christopher Curtis, "Chief Inspires Support," *Ottawa Citizen*, December 21, 2012, http://www.pressreader.com/canada/ottawa-citizen/20121221/283218735496368; "Chief Spence Out of Hospital after Ending 6-Week Hunger Strike," CTV News, January 24, 2013, https://www.ctvnews.ca/canada/chief-spence-out-of-hospital-after-ending-6-week-hunger-strike-1.1127449.

10. Tanya Talaga, "Wapekeka First Nation Feared Suicide Pact, Says They Were Denied Help," *Toronto Star*, January 19, 2017, https://www.thestar.com/news/canada/2017/01/19/wapekeka-first-nation-feared-suicide-pact-says-they-were-denied-help.html.

11. "Indigenous Leader Says He's Waiting for a National Strategy around Issue of Suicides," Global News, May 22, 2018, https://globalnews.ca/video/4223674/indigenous-leader-says-hes-waiting-for-a-national-strategy-around-issue-of-suicides.

12. Ibid.

13. Government of Canada (website), "Suicide Prevention," https://www.canada.ca/en/indigenous-services-canada/services/first-nations-inuit-health/health-promotion/suicide-prevention.html.

14. "Federal, Provincial and First Nations Leaders Taking Action on Health Transformation for First Nations in Nan Territory" (press release), Nishnawbe Aski Nation, November 27, 2017, http://www.nan.on.ca/article/november-17-2017-22522.asp.

15. Martin Luther King Jr., *Why We Can't Wait* (New York: Harper & Row, 1964), 119–20.

16. Dean J. Kotlowski, "Alcatraz, Wounded Knee, and Beyond: The Nixon and Ford Administrations Respond to Native American Protest," *Pacific Historical Review* 72, no. 2 (2003): 201–27, https://www-jstor-org.proxy3.library.mcgill.ca/stable/10.1525/phr.2003.72.2.201.

17. Troy R. Johnson, *Red Power: The Native Rights Movement* (New York: Infobase Publishing, 2009).

18. Troy R. Johnson, Duane Champagne, and Joane Nagel, "American Indian Activism and Transformation: Lessons from Alcatraz," in *American Indian Activism: Alcatraz to the Longest Walk*, ed. Troy Johnson, Joane Nagel, and Duane Champagne (Urbana: University of Illinois Press, 1997).

19. Troy R. Johnson and Joane Nagel, introduction to ibid., 1.

20. AKA Gallery (website), "Occupy Anishinabe Park 1974," http://akaartistrun.com/portfolio-item/occupy-anishinabe-park-1974/.

21. Interview with Richard Green, September 7, 2018.

22. Roy Cook, "'I Have a Dream for All God's Children': Martin Luther King Jr. Day," American Indian Source (website), http://americanindiansource.com/mlkechohawk.html; Matthew L. M. Fletcher, "A Short History of Indian Law in the Supreme Court," *Human Rights Magazine* 40, no. 4 (2014), https://www.americanbar.org/publications/human_rights_magazine_home/2014_vol_40/vol--40--no--1--tribal-sovereignty/short_history_of_indian_law.html.

23. Native American Rights Fund (website), "About Us," https://www.narf.org/about-us/.

24. Native American Rights Fund (website), "NARF Stands with Standing Rock," March 15, 2017, https://www.narf.org/narf-stands-standing-rock/.

25. Gregor Aisch and K. K. Rebecca Lai, "The Conflicts along 1,172 Miles of the Dakota Access Pipeline," *New York Times* (website), updated March 20, 2017, https://www.nytimes.com/

interactive/2016/11/23/us/dakota-access-pipeline-protest-map.html.

26. Stand with Standing Rock (website), "Camp Information: Oceti Sakowin," http://standwithstandingrock.net/oceti-sakowin/.

27. Chief Arvol Looking Horse, "Standing Rock Is Everywhere: One Year Later," *Guardian,* February 22, 2018, https://www.theguardian.com/environment/climate-consensus-97-per-cent/2018/feb/22/standing-rock-is-everywhere-one-year-later.

28. Tabitha Marshall, "Idle No More," in *The Canadian Encyclopedia Online,* April 12, 2013, https://www.thecanadianencyclopedia.ca/en/article/idle-no-more/.

29. Idle No More (website), "Idle No More Stands in Solidarity with Justice for Our Stolen Children Organizers," July 14, 2018, http://www.idlenomore.ca/justice_for_our_stolen_children.

30. Svein S. Andersen and Atle Midttun, "Conflict and Local Mobilization: The Alta Hydropower Project," *Acta Sociologica* 28, no. 4 (1985): 317–35, https://www.jstor.org/stable/4194584.

31. "5 Social Movements Resisting Regression in Latin America," Telesur, February 20, 2017, https://www.telesurtv.net/english/news/5-Social-Movements-Resisting-Repression-in-Latin-America-20170215-0042.html.

32. Angela Davis, *Freedom Is a Constant Struggle,* (Chicago: Haymarket Books, 2016), 121.

33. Interview with Helen Milroy.

34. Cindy Blackstock, "Jordan's Principle: Editorial update," *Paediatrics & Child Health,* 13, no. 7 (2008): 589–90.

35. Alex Soloducha, "Indigenous Family Receives Wheelchair Accessible House after Chief Applies for Access to Jordan's Principle," CBC News, December 12, 2017, https://www.cbc.ca/news/canada/manitoba/jordans-principle-could-have-prevented-wapekeka-first-nation-suicides-1.4134018.

36. Interview with Cindy Blackstock, *The House,* CBC Radio, December 1, 2017, http://www.cbc.ca/listen/shows/the-house/segment/15015697.

37. "Canada Fails to Grasp the 'Emergency' in First Nations Child Welfare: Canadian Human Rights Tribunal Finds Federal Government Non-Compliant with Relief Orders" (press release), First Nations Child and Family Caring Society of Canada, February 1, 2018, https://fncaringsociety.com/sites/default/files/Caring%20Society%20Press%20Release%202018%20CHRT%204.pdf.

38. Soloducha, "Indigenous Family Receives Wheelchair Accessible House."

39. Canadian Human Rights Tribunal, 2018 CHRT 4, 95, https://fncaringsociety.com/sites/default/files/2018%20CHRT%204.pdf.

40. Ibid., 96.

41. Andrew Kurjata, "How a Teddy Bear Received an Honorary Degree and Why His Work for Indigenous Children Still Isn't Done," CBC News, December 12, 2017, https://www.cbc.ca/news/canada/british-columbia/spirit-bear-jordans-principle-cindy-blackstock-1.4441093.

42. Blackstock interview, *The House*.

43. Murray Sinclair, speech to the judges of the Ontario Court of Justice, May 22, 2014.

44. Ibid., 7.

45. Ibid., 9.

46. Natan Obed, "The Challenge of Our Time" (lecture, Walrus Talks Arctic, Ottawa, September 2016), https://www.youtube.com/watch?v=YNomYzW7DdM.

47. Michele LeTourneau, "Territorial addictions and trauma treatment in the works," *Nunavut News*, February 23, 2018, https://nunavutnews.com/nunavut-news/territorial-addictions-trauma-treatment-works/.

48. Vicki Chartrand, "Broken System: Why Is a Quarter of Canada's Prison Population Indigenous?," *Conversation*, February 18, 2018, https://theconversation.com/broken-system-why-is-a-quarter-of-canadas-prison-population-indigenous-91562.

49. Jamil Malakieh, "Adult and Youth Correctional Statistics in Canada, 2016/2017," Statistics Canada (website), June 19, 2018, https://www150.statcan.gc.ca/n1/pub/85-002-x/2018001/article/54972-eng.htm.

50. Martin Luther King Jr., quoted in Davis, *Freedom Is a Constant Struggle*, 127.

51. Ibid., 53.

52. Nelson Mandela, *Long Walk to Freedom* (New York: Little, Brown, 1994), 544.

53. Barack Obama, Nelson Mandela Annual Lecture, Johannesburg, July 17, 2018, https://www.npr.org/2018/07/17/629862434/transcript-obamas-speech-at-the-2018-nelson-mandela-annual-lecture.

54. Sinclair, speech to judges of Ontario Court of Justice.

55. Thomas King, *The Truth About Stories* (Toronto: House of Anansi Press, 2003), 29, 60, 89, 119, 151, 167.

56. Ojibwe (website), "Basic Ojibwe Words and Phrases," http://www.ojibwe.org/home/pdf/Ojibwe_Beginner_Dictionary.pdf.

ACKNOWLEDGEMENTS

THIS BOOK WAS THE result of many voices coming together as one. Any fault in accuracy or facts are solely my own. So many people helped to bring this book together, and to those who I have missed in thanking, know that you are in my heart.

I am fortunate to know and be inspired by Nishnawbe Aski Nation Grand Chief Alvin Fiddler and his wife, teacher and educator Tesa Fiddler. Their deep knowledge, strong dedication, and resilience never falters, and from this many take great strength. We are proud to walk with you.

To Poplar Hill First Nation and to Wapekeka First Nation, to Wapekeka Chief Brennan Sainnawap and to the families of Amy Owen, Kanina Sue Turtle, Jolynn Winter, Chantell Fox, Alayna Moose, Jenera

Roundsky, and Jeannie Grace Brown: my sincere condolences. Your strength is second to none.

Elder Sam Achneepineskum, your daily dose of encouragement, kind words, and humour have kept me grounded, connected. Much manajiwin. Our journey continues. To your sister Anna Betty Achneepineskum: you are a warrior, you pave the way. Never stop.

Ontario MPP Sol Mamakwa, John Cutfeet, Ovide Mercredi, and Dr. Michael Kirlew, your voices have raised this book. You seek justice for our children. Your work brings hope.

For those of us who are descendants of residential school survivors, it is impossible to put into words the debt we owe Senator Murray Sinclair. He embodies our Grandfathers' teachings. We would be lost without his words, his work, his keen eye, and his great sense of debwewin.

Lee Maracle, you paved the way and we wouldn't be here without your strength, support, and gentle nudges, pointing us to where we need to be.

I am profoundly grateful to Natan Obed for always generously, and at a moment's notice, extending a hand in friendship and in teachings. You are a gifted leader, an educator, and a truth teller. The Inuit Tapiriit Kanatami National Inuit

Suicide Prevention Strategy is a path forward. Our Inuit brothers and sisters lead the way. To Adam Akpik, thank you for your time and tour of Iqaluit.

Mushkegowuk Grand Chief Jonathan Solomon, your words and endless dedication to the youth is a shining example of strength. To Ed Metatawabin and Mike Metatawabin, your lives, words, and your work teach us all. You never give up in your relentless search for justice and we thank you for this.

Hayden King, chi-miigwech for introducing me to Alan Corbiere; and Alan, I am honoured to know you and am grateful for all of your advice.

Michael Heintzman, again, I would be lost without your unwavering support and willingness to help. I've said it before, I'll say it again: you are the best at what you do. To Luke Hunter, thank you for the Treaty No. 9 interpretations and for your generous assistance. To Derek Fox, miigwech for the book and for the devoted work you continue to do with youth.

To my House of Anansi family: Laura Meyer, Maria Golikova, Alexandra Trnka, Alysia Shewchuk, Laura Brady, Irina Malakhova, Matt Williams, and Sarah MacLachlan. We have moved a mountain and we have done this together. Sarah, thank you for keeping your eye on the ball. Peter Norman and

Gillian Watts, you have done the heavy lifting at the eleventh hour. Many thanks.

To my editor, Janie Yoon: this book would not have happened if it weren't for you. You have my deep respect, love, and sincere appreciation. You pulled me through the dark patches and sat with me, every step of the way. You sacrificed so much of your time and blessed this manuscript with your wisdom. These Massey Lectures are truly the result of a great partnership. I am honoured to be your friend.

To my *Toronto Star* family, my home base: I couldn't have done this without the support of the *Star* newsroom. I'm blessed to work with Lynn McAuley, the greatest narrative editor around. Irene Gentle, thank you for believing in your staff. To John Honderich, the *Star* family is a beautiful one and we do great things. We are a paper for the people and will continue to be that voice. To my Atkinson Foundation family, to Colette Murphy and Jenn Miller: thank you for all you do to make the world a more equitable place.

To Helen Milroy and Rose LeMay, you both lead by example. The Creator brought you both into my life for a reason. I am honoured to have received your guidance.

· ACKNOWLEDGEMENTS ·

Leslie Bonshor, I am so happy you reached out and told me that I needed to meet with you. As always, you were right. Keep going with your work, and miigwech for introducing me to the Stó:lō Nation. Maggie Pettis, your kind heart heals many.

To the staff at the Wabano Centre: I am in awe of what you do and inspired by the incredible team of women leading the way. To Jack Hicks, thank you for your research and time.

To Philip Coulter and Greg Kelly, you have given me this great opportunity and have stood solidly behind me — miigwech. Stuart Coxe, you've got the vision and always the sound advice.

To Cindy Blackstock, as always, you guide us. I could not do this without the unrelenting work of the First Nations Family and Caring Society. Riley Yesno, you are the future. You will do great things and I'm honoured to be cheering you on. Thank you to Evan Grant and Alison Grant for helping me with research.

As always, my friends, family, and loved ones have given me immeasurable support and I have asked a lot of you during this last year.

Dirk Huyer, thank you for listening, and for the conversations on the determinants of health, and for being there.

Michelle Shephard, your strength and laughter keep me whole. Patty Winsa, Rita Daly, Justine Keyserlingk, Chantelle Bryson — thank you.

To my mother, Sheila Van Sluytman: you have been the great influence in my life and you have always been my hero, an example of how to lead and to love. To my brother, Yuri, and to Maureen, Joseph, and Thomas: thank you for sharing so much. To my late sister, Donna: I carry you with me. To my grandmother Margaret, to my uncles Maurice and Bill, to my Aunt Cheryl, and to my late Uncle Alvie — our spirits intertwine. To all my relations, we are resilience.

To my children, William and Natasha: I have asked so much of you and you have always, always been there for a hug, a good poke, and constant laughter. Know you are always loved and that you come from strength. I could not do any of this without you.

My true hope is that *All Our Relations* instills pride and belonging in Indigenous youth and that they see that they are part of the greater continuum. They will lead us on the path forward.

Qamaniittuaq, Nunavut
September 2018

INDEX

(THE CBC MASSEY LECTURES SERIES)

Reset
Ronald J. Deibert
978-1-4870-0805-5 (CAN)
978-1-4870-0808-6 (U.S.)

Power Shift
Sally Armstrong
978-1-4870-0679-2 (CAN)
978-1-4870-0682-2 (U.S.)

In Search of a Better World
Payam Akhavan
978-1-4870-0200-8 (CAN)
978-1-4870-0339-5 (U.S.)

Therefore Choose Life
George Wald
978-1-4870-0320-3 (CAN)
978-1-4870-0338-8 (U.S.)

The Return of History
Jennifer Welsh
978-1-4870-0242-8

History's People
Margaret MacMillan
978-1-4870-0137-7

Belonging
Adrienne Clarkson
978-1-77089-837-0 (CAN)
978-1-77089-838-7 (U.S)

Blood
Lawrence Hill
978-1-77089-322-1 (CAN)
978-1-77089-323-8 (U.S.)

The Universe Within
Neil Turok
978-1-77089-015-2 (CAN)
978-1-77089-017-6 (U.S.)

Winter
Adam Gopnik
978-0-88784-974-9 (CAN)
978-0-88784-975-6 (U.S.)

Player One
Douglas Coupland
978-0-88784-972-5 (CAN)
978-0-88784-968-8 (U.S.)

The Wayfinders
Wade Davis
978-0-88784-842-1 (CAN)
978-0-88784-766-0 (U.S.)

Payback
Margaret Atwood
978-0-88784-810-0 (CAN)
978-0-88784-800-1 (U.S.)

The City of Words
Alberto Manguel
978-0-88784-763-9

More Lost Massey Lectures
Bernie Lucht, ed.
978-0-88784-801-8

The Lost Massey Lectures
Bernie Lucht, ed.
978-0-88784-217-7

The Ethical Imagination
Margaret Somerville
978-0-88784-747-9

Race Against Time
Stephen Lewis
978-0-88784-753-0

A Short History of Progress
Ronald Wright
978-0-88784-706-6

Available in fine bookstores and at www.houseofanansi.com